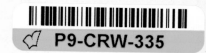

Praise for *Up for the Fight*

"Receiving a cancer diagnosis can be a life-altering, scary moment. Due to the ever-increasing complexity of modern medicine, patients are often faced with the challenging task of navigating between multiple doctors, understanding a rapidly changing treatment landscape, and dealing with the physical and emotional burdens that accompany a diagnosis. The right path is not always obvious and taking a wrong turn can sometimes lead to disastrous results. Unfortunately, resources to help guide patients are often scattered, outdated, or, at worst, wrong. Bill C. Potts has created an incredible tool for families, caregivers, and patients to navigate the battle against cancer. By using his years of experience as a guide, Bill provides unique and invaluable insight into what it took to win his own battle. I hope that every new cancer patient has an opportunity to read this incredible book and use it as a resource to beat cancer."

DR. NATHAN FOWLER, Professor of Medicine, MD Anderson Cancer Center, Houston, TX; Chief Medical Officer, BostonGene; Co-Founder, Halo House Foundation

"As an oncologist treating many cancer patients, including Bill C. Potts, I am grateful that Bill wrote this book and will recommend it to those dealing with cancer. It provides information that patients and their families will find practical and helpful, from the perspective of a very experienced patient."

DR. ERNESTO AYALA, hematologist and oncologist, Mayo Clinic, Jacksonville, FL

"I've worked closely with multiple myeloma patients for more than a decade, and I have seen firsthand how incredibly difficult it is for patients when they first hear the words, 'You have cancer.' Patients and their loved ones then start on a journey to navigate their disease so that they can all become core members of the care team. *Up for the Fight* provides solid, specific advice to help patients know what to do as they ride this bumpy road. I highly recommend this incredibly useful and easy-to-read book to anyone going through the cancer journey. It provides great insights on how to best manage the diagnosis, and offers tips from the start to finish of treatment. I only wish this book had been written when I started my own cancer journey."

JANE HOFFMANN, Senior Director, Events and Partnerships, Multiple Myeloma Research Foundation; cancer survivor

"Supporting my dad through his cancer journey was incredibly important to me. *Up for the Fight* is an informative resource that provides family members with the tools they need to support their loved one through the cancer journey."

MEG NOLTE, daughter of a cancer survivor

How to Advocate for Yourself as
You Battle Cancer
from a Five-Time Survivor

BILL C. POTTS

UP FOR THE FIGHT

PAGE TWO

Copyright © 2022 by Bill C. Potts

All rights reserved. No part of this book may be reproduced,
stored in a retrieval system or transmitted, in any form or by any
means, without the prior written consent of the publisher or a
licence from The Canadian Copyright Licensing Agency (Access
Copyright). For a copyright licence, visit accesscopyright.ca
or call toll free to 1-800-893-5777.

Some names and identifying details have been changed
to protect the privacy of individuals.

This book is not intended as a substitute for the medical
advice of physicians. The reader should regularly consult
a physician in matters relating to his/her/their health
and particularly with respect to any symptoms that may
require diagnosis or medical attention.

Cataloguing in publication information is
available from Library and Archives Canada.
ISBN 978-1-77458-168-1 (paperback)
ISBN 978-1-77458-169-8 (ebook)
ISBN 978-1-77458-261-9 (audiobook)

Page Two
pagetwo.com

Edited by Amanda Lewis
Copyedited by Shyla Seller
Proofread by Alison Strobel
Cover design by Taysia Louie
Interior design by Fiona Lee
Printed and bound in Canada by Friesens
Distributed in Canada by Raincoast Books
Distributed in the US and internationally by Macmillan

22 23 24 25 26   5 4 3 2 1

billcpotts.com

To my amazing family, who has supported me throughout this long and continuing journey. My soulmate and wife, Kim, has been my rock and support. My three kids, Nick, Sarah, and Anna, have been incredible. Their hugs, popsicles, calls, and visits mean the world to me. My sweet dog, Pippa, has been by my side non-stop. She is a great listener!

To my mom, Barbara, who taught me how to fight by winning her own brutal battle with cancer. To my late dad, Tom Potts, who always encouraged his kids to write— and inspired me with his own cancer fight.

To the thousands of brave, tough kids and adults I met at Clearwater Marine Aquarium. The people in wheelchairs, those with prosthetic limbs, the wounded warriors, the cancer patients, and all those who were up for the fight in the face of adversity. You inspire me.

And to the millions of cancer patients and their families fighting their battles, and to all the health care professionals fighting valiantly for them!

CONTENTS

Own your cancer journey.
Your life depends on it.

FOREWORD

IT HAS been over ten years since I first met Bill in the lymphoma clinic at MD Anderson Cancer Center. I was the advanced practice nurse on Bill's cancer care team and worked closely with Dr. Nathan Fowler, a specialist in the lymphoma clinic.

Bill had an interesting story. He'd been previously diagnosed with thyroid cancer, and his biopsy was showing a new primary, also known as a completely different kind of cancer. This new cancer might have been mistreated had he not advocated so well for himself.

Bill appeared cool, calm, and collected that day, though I can only imagine what he must have been feeling and experiencing beneath the surface. He shared his cancer story, which is such an important part of the initial visit. Together we came up with a plan. We also established a patient-nurse relationship based on sharing, listening, and supporting, which has turned into a friendship that I'm grateful to have.

Bill followed the plan that Dr. Fowler set for him. One unforgettable day, we were able to tell him, "You're in a remission. No cancer was seen on the scans."

What many people don't realize is that the hardest part. of having cancer often starts once the treatment and constant clinic visits end. When the health care team has been holding your hand throughout the treatment, it can feel like they're letting go and leaving you to face the journey ahead on your own. Bill was great about staying in touch and keeping us informed about his recovery and healing. He shared with us that he wanted to complete IRONMAN Texas after he went into remission. Not only did he stay in touch with us, he invited Dr. Fowler and me to meet him at the IRONMAN finish line!

It was over 100 degrees in Houston that day and many athletes were struggling on the course, but Bill made it to the finish line and gave us a big ol' hug as he crossed. I told him, "You're amazing! Now I have to do a triathlon!" Right at that moment, race day caught up with him and he got wobbly, his knees started to shake, and someone scooped him up with a wheelchair and ran him to the medical tent where he recovered with IV fluids. I was hoping he'd forget what I said. But no, he called me the next day and said, "Liz! I'll never forget what you said!"

The point is, Bill is an incredibly inspiring human and he made an impression on me from the very first day. I went on to complete seven triathlons while raising money for the Leukemia and Lymphoma Society.

Bill managed his cancer journey with vulnerability, wholeheartedness, courage, and faith. He's written this book using these same qualities, and has used his gifts of inspiration and discipline to outline all the most important points to help many people along their journey.

I hope you are as inspired by Bill as I have been, and I wish you well on your journey.

ELIZABETH SORENSEN
Advanced Practice Nurse at MD *Anderson Cancer Center, Houston, Texas, 2006-2013*

INTRODUCTION

O N SEPTEMBER 17, 2020, I woke up sobbing in the recovery room at the Mayo Clinic in Jacksonville, Florida. I had just gone through surgery to remove a painful and cancerous tumor from my groin area. I had gone into the surgery scared but stoic and confident. I had awoken to an emotional breakdown.

As the tears flowed, Jen Green, the nurse sitting by my side, reached down, held my hand, and asked me, "Bill, what is wrong?"

The words that came out of my mouth astonished both of us.

"Jen, I am thinking about giving up the cancer fight. Maybe it is time to throw in the towel."

Then I told her my story: "This is the sixth time I have been diagnosed with cancer and my fifth cancer surgery. This is the fourth time I have had lymphoma, after only eleven months in remission. Two months ago, I was diagnosed with prostate cancer, too. So, now I have two cancers at the same time. And my type of lymphoma is incurable and will come back. This is on top of the thyroid cancer I had twenty years ago."

I have had a very fulfilling life since my initial cancer diagnosis. My cancer has driven me to try and accomplish a lot, as fast as I could. It changed my priorities.

I have helped raise three awesome kids, and am in an amazing marriage. I have had a successful career in marketing. I have worked at IRONMAN, am an IRONMAN athlete, have run marathons, and have even run up the Empire State Building. I spent the past four-plus years in a job I loved, at Clearwater Marine Aquarium. A job with a deep purpose, where I was able to meet thousands of kids and adults with physical and emotional challenges. I watched them be inspired and changed just by meeting Winter, the dolphin. I was BFFs with Hope, the dolphin, with whom I played hide and seek each morning. The people who I met were inspired in turn, by the care and love of the amazing aquarium team who rescued, rehabilitated, and released marine life. Each day at the aquarium, I had the opportunity to help change lives, and I was proud of the work I did there. I worked to prove to my family that anything is possible. That no matter what happens to you—with hard work, a positive attitude, and a great support team—big goals can be accomplished.

"But," I finally paused to take a breath. "I know what is coming with the cancer treatment . . . and I don't like it."

Jen called the Mayo pastor, Tanya, who had been with me just prior to the surgery. Tanya listened as I told my story. I started asking her questions about why she worked at Mayo Clinic with patients like me.

Her powerful answers helped me reconnect with my *why*. Why I needed to fight cancer again, and beat it: For my family and friends, to inspire others, for the non-profit clients at my marketing agency, to make God proud.

AN HOUR after my meltdown began, I reconnected with my purpose. I was ready and up for the fight. I believe that miracles happen—and my change of heart was itself a miracle.

Tanya wrapped up our chat with the following comment. "Bill, your story is unique. You should write a book and share with others what you have learned through your journey. Use your pain for the purpose of helping others."

This is that book.

CANCER, TO quote author John Green, is a civil war. Cancer is a part of me. A bad part. It is trying to kill the good part of me. So, it is the good me fighting the bad me. Thus, "battling" cancer. A civil war.

Let's be up front. I hate cancer. I am not a doctor, but a cancer veteran. A survivor. You have to be a survivor in order to really understand how to battle cancer. For example, I am an avid runner. What is some of the best advice I have given runners doing their first 5k? Double-knot your shoelaces. This is insight which can only be provided by someone who has experienced their shoelaces coming untied in a race.

This book is like that insight, but for cancer.

UP FOR THE FIGHT is cancer uncut, the real story. While writing this book, I went through fourteen chemotherapy and immunotherapy treatments for my lymphoma, a blood cancer, as well as multiple surgeries, two minor, one major. I had a surgical biopsy of my prostate, related to my prostate cancer. I wrote while grinding through physical and emotional pain. It was not easy. There were days and weeks when I was too sick to write. Reliving what I had been through, was going through, was painful. But this book has provided me great purpose. A reason to get up, head to our garage apartment, write and share what I learned. I wrote it while in relative isolation, in a bubble, as the beatdown of my immune system from chemotherapy and the risk of getting COVID-19 or a flu or cold prevented me from being around many people.

I know the cancer issues. I have been through the journey—a lot. Five times surviving. Number six in progress. Number seven likely just a few years away.

IF YOU have been diagnosed with cancer, you are in the Cancer Club. Like being a marathoner or an IRONMAN, you will always be in that club. Your family and friends will be in this club, too.

As a long-time member of the Cancer Club, I have learned how to advocate for myself. I am 100 percent certain that had I not advocated for myself, I would not be alive to write this book.

The biggest problem I've had during my twenty-year cancer journey? Learning from trial and error what works, every step of the way. There was no guide on what to expect—physically, mentally, emotionally. I wish I had read a book like this at the start of my journey, but none existed. I have been surprised a thousand times, with head-spinning stuff. Just having some idea of what to expect would have made a positive difference for me and my family.

THIS BOOK is not a critique of the current medical system. Modern medicine has saved me five times so far, and I have been fortunate to be treated at two of the best cancer clinics in the US, MD Anderson Cancer Center in Houston and the Mayo Clinic (Jacksonville campus).

What this book will do is guide you through the cancer journey—from first steps when getting the news, to tests you may get to stage it; what types of treatment to expect; and how to ace your treatment days, manage side effects, and anticipate the unexpected. Also, I've included tips on dealing with the mental and emotional side of the journey, which can be as hard or harder than the treatment itself.

If you read only two chapters, please read Chapters 4 and 5. They will offer suggestions on how to work within the medical system, advocating for yourself on your own cancer journey, as well as how to pick a care team. In my favorite chapter, Chapter 14, you will hear from my family about their tips for family members on the journey, followed by advice for the friends of cancer patients. Chapter 7, on the business of cancer, offers practical insights on your options for fighting cancer. I also address the possibility of dying (Chapter 13), and offer insight on how cancer impacts you after the treatment is finished (Chapter 15). I know it's hard to fathom, but going through the cancer journey may change your life and the lives of those around you in a positive way.

If you are reading this book, you or someone you know has been given the tough news. You are in the Cancer Club. Remember, you are not alone. There are not only millions of others in your same situation, but many people and organizations who will support you along the way.

I wrote this book with two simple goals. One, to help you learn from my mistakes. Two, to tell you what most doctors can't tell you about fighting cancer, from the perspective of the cancer patient.

Some of my favorite motivational lessons:

- Remind yourself every day of the reasons you are fighting. Every day. This is a great motivational tool.

- Run your cancer journey like it is a race. Break it into small goals, and celebrate these goals along the way until you finish.

- Celebrate each step of the journey. First treatment— booyah! Halfway through treatment—booyah! Finish treatment—ring the bell!

- Celebrate birthdays, anniversaries, and other occasions that happen during your journey—with gusto!

- Celebrate accomplishments of your friends and family during your journey—with gusto!

- Tell your family and friends you love them.

1

THE TOUGH NEWS

A S OF the writing of this book, I have been in the Cancer Club for twenty years. I have been told I have cancer seven times. One diagnosis was wrong, but six, unfortunately, were right.

My journey started when I was forty-one years old, in 2002. I was diagnosed with thyroid cancer. The news came out of nowhere. I was totally unprepared for what lay ahead. At the time, I had been married ten years to my wife, Kim, and was the father of four-year-old twin girls, Sarah and Anna, and a seven-year-old son, Nick.

The thyroid cancer was cured, but I received the bad news again in 2003 (incorrectly, a return of the thyroid cancer), 2008 (lymphoma), 2014 (lymphoma), 2019 (lymphoma), and 2020 (lymphoma plus prostate cancer). My lymphoma is incurable, and we are already planning how to handle it when it comes back.

Starting the fight
. . . .

I had just come back from completing IRONMAN 70.3 Cancún, in 2008, when I noticed a lump below my right ear. Given my scare with thyroid cancer, I immediately went to my primary care physician, who referred me to an ear, nose, and throat doctor. This doctor conducted surgery to remove what at the time was thought to be a harmless infected parotid gland. Later, I went to the same doctor's office to have thirteen staples removed from the surgical incision.

After he removed my staples, the doctor read out loud from the biopsy report. About halfway through the report, he read that the gland was not an infected gland, but a cancerous lymph node—diagnosed as lymphoma.

Incredibly, he just kept reading, not even paying attention to me!

I stopped him and asked him to re-read the part about cancer. He did and promptly told me I needed to leave his office, as he did not handle cancer patients. He handed me the biopsy report and asked his receptionist to give me the business card of an oncologist across the street. Three minutes after learning I had lymphoma, I was already out of his office, without understanding what lymphoma was or what the diagnosis meant. What a stressful way to start my lymphoma battle! My head was spinning.

Cancer sucks

Having cancer sucks in so many ways. Like really, really sucks. After being diagnosed, you may be thinking:

- Why me?

- I am busy and don't have time for cancer.

- I didn't do anything to deserve cancer.

Cancer impacts everyone **in a unique way.**

- What do I do about work and my career?

- What about my other responsibilities?

- What about my vacation?

- How much will this cost?

- I just retired . . . now this?

- What happens to my family if I die?

- Life was going great—and now cancer is messing it up.

- How will my family handle my going through treatment?

- What about the place I volunteer? Who will take over?

- But I just got engaged/married/had a baby.

- I don't want to let my team down, at work or play.

Feelings of dread, anguish, hopelessness, fear, sadness, anxiety, and many others will all jumble together inside you. I live it. I get it. We can all choose to be consumed by these types of emotions, but we can also try to be positive. That doesn't mean you won't have a lot of negative feelings come and go. That is natural. Those feelings will happen. But you need to harness those feelings and work as hard as you can to have a positive attitude as often as you can.

Why? A good attitude can make a positive difference in many ways. A good attitude will:

- Make a positive impact on your care team. I have seen this firsthand. The grumpy patient's attitude may have an unwittingly negative impact on their caregivers. It is hard to quantify, but attitudes are contagious.

- Make a difference with your family and friends. It is with 100 percent certainty that they will want to interact with you more if you are positive. We all are this way—and may not realize it—but we naturally avoid negativity, if we can. As a cancer patient, you need all the family and social support you can get!

- Help you inspire others. I have heard this a thousand times: "Bill, it is amazing that you continue to have a great attitude through your treatment. It is inspiring and makes my problems feel small. Your attitude gives me perspective."

- Improve your journey. I don't know the science behind it, but I believe the less stress you have, combined with a good or positive attitude, can help your body heal better. I don't want to mislead you. A lot has to happen and go right to beat cancer. Attitude is only one piece of it; it alone cannot heal you.

Understand, too, that at times the weight of it all makes it impossible to be positive. This is true of all cancer patients at some point in their journey. For others, this is true for the entirety of their journey. Cancer impacts everyone in a unique way. There is no right or wrong. If you cannot muster a good or positive attitude, give yourself grace. Sadness and anxiety are so common that antidepressant and anti-anxiety medications are often prescribed to cancer patients.

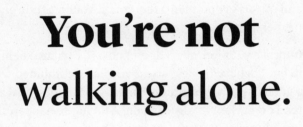

You're not
walking alone.

Hearing the news

I lost it when I first learned I had cancer. I felt sick and had to run to the bathroom. I was rattled to the core. Hearing the words "you have cancer" immediately turns your life upside down. I call the challenge of thinking clearly after a diagnosis the *cancer fog*. Your thinking is hazy and slow. Your first instinct is to panic. Don't. Know there is a *lot* of support to help you in your journey. You're not walking alone.

You are scared, nervous, and have a million things to think about—not just your cancer, but life in general. You may be thinking for the first time about the possibility of dying. On top of this, you have a thousand things to manage about your cancer: where to go, scheduling appointments, work issues, family issues. It is a lot. I was lost at first, but after a few days started pulling it together.

There is no shortcut to handling the emotions that arise following a cancer diagnosis. You will go through some of the stages of grief. At first, I was in shock and in disbelief, then quite mad, then very sad, and then I finally got to acceptance, where I needed to be. I recommend right up front getting professional outside help in the form of therapists, psychiatrists, faith leaders like a pastor or rabbi, or support groups. Understand that it is 100 percent OK not to be OK—and no one expects you to be 100 percent OK. *No one* is ever 100 percent OK.

Once you get the news, your priorities immediately shift to beating cancer. The seriousness of being in the Cancer Club cannot be understated.

Whatever cancer you are diagnosed with, you will quickly need to pick and visit with specialists. Focus and speed really become important. According to medical research, the first four weeks after many initial cancer diagnoses are critical, and how critical varies depending on the type of cancer. The point here is—get moving on it! Most cancer centers will work as fast as they can to get you in to see them. Chapter 5 provides guidance on how to select the best cancer care team.

You can live to be a hundred years old and still be impacted by being a member of the Cancer Club. It's a lifetime membership.

As a part of this club, you will also see the world and life in a wonderful new way. Mentally and emotionally, you will be different. The big things that stressed you become small things and the small things that stressed you go away. It is like taking off blinders you didn't know you were wearing; you get a clarity and perspective about life you did not have before. This is something you experience only when fighting a battle of life and death. This new perspective may change the trajectory of your life.

Another blessing is the strengthening of faith or spirituality. The chance of dying at a young age woke me up to the importance of God and faith. I lean into my Christian faith now more than ever. I pray often for wisdom to make the right decisions about my treatment. It has worked!

The emotions of cancer are not just confined to you; they impact your loved ones. My wife took it in stride in 2002 and, thankfully, unlike me, did not overreact. She knew that her role was to be strong for me and our three young kids. They were too young to understand exactly what was going on, but were perceptive enough to know something was very wrong with their dad.

2

THE EMOTIONAL ASPECT

HERE IS the biggest tip for grounding yourself at the start of your cancer journey: *Find your whys*. Identify the reasons why you want to fight the battle and win. It could be family, friends, goals you want to accomplish, work. Once you identify the reasons you want to fight to beat cancer—write them down. These whys are super important and will guide you throughout your journey. Your cancer whys become your "get up and go."

The emotions of cancer patients run like a roller coaster, up and down and around the bend. Except you can't see or know what is around the corner. What hill or trough is next? Your emotions can run wild, impossible to predict.

Just yesterday, out of the blue, I had a rough day physically and emotionally. I woke up in pain, sad and blue, with no real explanation for it. I didn't want to be around people; I needed time alone. The day before, I had been calm and happy. Tomorrow, who knows.

This is the life of a cancer patient.

I am told all the time that people respond well to my positive attitude. They do. I am just wired positive by nature. But sometimes, because of my cancer, I fake it.

Why? Because there are many times when you just don't want to talk or even think about cancer. You want to get away from the topic. That is one reason I limit who even knows about my cancer.

When someone asks me how I am, many times I answer with a simple, "I am great. Getting through it." That will suffice and end that direction of the conversation. When pushed, I will update them on my status. "I am halfway through my chemo." "I am finished with my treatment." "I am getting stronger by the day."

With close friends, I open up and give them a bit more of the uncut version. "The chemo is brutal. I feel rough but am sleeping a lot." "I am having a hard day." But I rarely if ever reveal much detail to my friends. If I need to share how I really feel, a support group is a great place to do it, as they will understand my experiences. It is impossible to know what it feels like to be a cancer patient unless you are in the Cancer Club. All will respect your decision to seek outside support.

The seasons

The cancer journey has many seasons. There is a pattern, a cadence. After the initial shock of the diagnosis, you begin the fall season. The start of treatment, when the job of beating cancer begins in earnest. During this season, you are more likely to be happy to get the treatment going and get into the routine. The colors are still bright. The air fresh. You are on the journey and making progress. Your mood may be pretty good.

Like with the actual seasons, winter sneaks up on you. All of a sudden, the tone shifts a bit. The days are shorter,

Find your whys.
Identify the reasons
why you want to fight
the battle and win.

the nights longer, and while you are going through treatment, it is starting to get a bit old. The treatment is cumulative, so your body is feeling its impact even more. Anxious excitement felt at the beginning of the journey turns to fatigue. Fatigue with the body and mind. The days drag. Time slows down. You sleep more. You may become more irritable. You dread heading to treatment. Just one season ago, you were ready to get started. It's like switching to the night shift after working the day shift. It can become hard just to walk in the door for treatment. This is completely normal.

Spring comes just in time. Your mood brightens like it does when the flowers bloom outside. You have made it halfway through your treatment and you are counting down to the end. You have likely had a "halfway through treatment" scan, and if the results are good, you are feeling positive. Now, instead of dreading treatment, you become happy to go because you can finally see the finish line!

Summer! This season starts when you are finished with treatment and the scans give you good news. Your mood brightens even more than it did with the spring. Glorious summer is here. You worry less. Soon, cancer won't be the center of your life. Now you can put your focus on other things.

The length of each season will vary depending on your treatment and progress. I have had short winters and very long winters. I have had a summer of six-and-a-half years and one of eleven months.

I know the seasons will change, but they do not always progress in that exact order. Sometimes, you will go from fall to winter to spring and back to winter again. It depends on how effective your treatment is. In my case, with two cancers to manage at the same time, my seasons get stretched. I hope to get to summer—it may just take me a bit longer.

The job mindset

Treat the cancer journey like it is your job. It is! At a job, you would have goals. You would have a list of next steps. You would have a calendar of events. You would prepare online, speak with people, and read books to gather information.

Here's an example: We recently renovated our living room and dining room. My wife treated the renovations like a job. She was on top of it with the contractors: Setting goals, managing timetables, making changes in real time as needed. She got it done on schedule, which was great, as I could not be in the house when the workers were there. Their work was great too. We love it!

The more you apply this job mindset to getting well, the more you will engage. All this means *you* are taking charge of your cancer. Taking charge should help reduce your anxiety. Own it; manage it. Taking charge and advocating for yourself helps you disconnect a bit from the emotions. Some of this will happen naturally, and is your mind's way of protecting you. But the mindset that it is your *job* to beat cancer really changes your perspective.

3

COMMUNICATING THE TOUGH NEWS

NOW THAT you are in the Cancer Club, how do you communicate with others about your health?

First of all, upon initial diagnosis—limit who you tell, for three reasons.

1 You need to process the news first—and this takes some time. You don't need others calling and visiting you yet. You will find early on that everyone will want to tell you a cancer story, or recommend a doctor, a diet, or a treatment. Avoid these distractions by limiting who you tell.

2 Sometimes the initial diagnosis needs confirmation or is incorrect.

3 You need to focus on yourself and your plan. You don't need to handle the emotions of others as you map out next steps.

Don't post anything about your cancer on social media. Up until the marketing for the release of the book, many of the people I know did not know I have cancer. This is on purpose.

There are work issues at play. Future employers will likely check you out on social media. Do you really want your future employer to know about your cancer? How

Pause, and then
be deliberate
as to who you share
the news with.

much do you want your employer to know about your diagnosis, if, for example, you get considered for a promotion?

Limit talking about it at work. Of course, your boss may need to know. Human Resources may need to know—but other than that, there are limited benefits in discussing your diagnosis at work. However, if people need to know to help keep you safe or if you need their support and encouragement, addressing it may be worthwhile.

In the US, at work, your health is confidential and protected under federal law (i.e., in many cases, it is illegal for your boss to disclose your cancer to others). If in doubt about what to do, a labor attorney can provide guidance, and, if needed, work with you on a plan to allow you to not work so that you can recover, using disability insurance, if you have it.

People at work may know or need to know, depending on your circumstances (e.g., if you lose your hair or are immunocompromised). Perhaps working from home is an option, or having a private office, or staggering your hours. Maybe you can skip big in-person meetings in the office and do video calls instead. Maybe staff can wear surgical masks around you. The COVID-19 pandemic has highlighted different ways of working to protect people's health, and this can benefit cancer patients. Practicing physical distancing to protect an immunocompromised co-worker is becoming more common.

I do tell my close friends and relatives. But I wait until the diagnosis is confirmed and the treatment plan developed. You will want them to know, because you will need their support throughout your journey. But I preface these discussions with, "this is private information, not meant to be shared, including on social media." Tell them via phone, not text or social media.

Whatever approach you follow, be sure to take a deep breath when getting the tough news. Pause, and then be deliberate as to who you share the news with.

The journey is hard. Like a great story, the plot will have many twists and turns.

4

TAKE CHARGE!

MADE A mistake with my first cancer, my thyroid cancer, and that mistake may yet cost me my life.

I listened to my then–primary care physician's recommendation on who to see for my surgery and for my cancer treatment. I did not get a second opinion.

The recommended oncologists were a small, local operation (two doctors), for-profit, and happy to have me as a customer. After a five-hour surgery, where my thyroid gland was completely removed, the oncologist prescribed radioactive iodine therapy to kill any remaining cancer cells. I checked into a room in a remote area of a hospital and was given a radioactive pill, delivered to me in a big lead container, to kill any remnants of my thyroid cancer. The pill was the same type of radiation released when the nuclear power plant in Chernobyl melted down: iodine-131.

I was in the hospital in total isolation for days. The staff would only talk to me through a window or on the phone. I was there until a Geiger counter measured my radioactivity to be within legal limits and therefore determined it was safe enough for me to leave the hospital.

Everything I was wearing or touched while in the hospital was put into a red hazard bag and destroyed. I even had to throw away my clothes, the glasses I had worn, the hospital phone, and the small radio I had taken into the room with me.

While I could leave the hospital, I was not allowed to be near my young kids for a couple of weeks. THAT is how much radiation I was given.

The good news is that it worked and cured my thyroid cancer.

Six months later, after a standard follow-up scan, these same doctors recommended I go through radioactive iodine therapy again. Holy cow! That did not make any sense to me, as I did not even have a thyroid, or any remnants left to destroy. I was still adapting to the thyroid replacement medications they had given me. I was even gaining a lot of weight.

Only then did I start to ask questions. I decided to go to the MD Anderson Cancer Center in Houston, Texas, for a second opinion. MD Anderson is what I call a high-volume cancer center. They specialize in cancer care. They got me in quickly. After their own scan of my neck, MD Anderson disagreed with the need for me to get any further radiation. In fact, they were concerned about the amount I had already been given and even whether my whole thyroid should have come out.

You will read later about my second and third cancers; we will never know for certain their causes, but I have now had lymphoma four times and prostate cancer once, all AFTER my thyroid cancer treatment. I had first been exposed to radiation during my work at a hospital in college, in the department of nuclear medicine. That radiation likely contributed to my thyroid cancer. That, combined with my radioactive iodine therapy, has made

If you have not planned to get a second opinion—**please consider getting one.**

me a petri dish for cancer. I would likely be dead already if I had not gotten a second opinion, and instead received that second dose of iodine-131.

One of my newer cancers may still kill me, however. Not getting a second opinion is a major reason I wrote this book, so others don't make the same mistake that I made.

If you have not planned to get a second opinion—please consider getting one. The excuses I've heard from patients for not getting a second opinion include: "I like my doctor, he (or she) is so nice." "My doctor is close to where I live." "My doctor treats my neighbor." "My doctor gets great reviews." "I trust my doctor." That may all be true—and this person or team may become your cancer doctor—but for heaven's sake, get a second opinion!

Getting a second opinion, though, is just one part of the biggest cancer lesson.

The biggest cancer lesson

Advocate for yourself. Take charge of your cancer journey. It is YOUR life. YOU must OWN it. No one else. No one! Dammit! Listen!

The idea that you, the patient, own your journey to recovery may be counterintuitive. Many generations have been taught that the doctor or care team owns your journey. The care team is critical, and you should listen to them, but only YOU can best advocate for yourself. They are not you! You know you. You know your body; you know how you feel physically, mentally, emotionally. Your care team will listen to you and respect you owning your journey.

Some people embrace owning their cancer journey and others don't. Pretty, pretty, pretty please—don't be the old me—not owning my journey. Be the new me, owning and being involved every step of the way.

Please advocate for yourself! It is worth the effort!

5

THE CARE TEAM

AFTER YOU receive the initial cancer diagnosis, time seems to slow down. Beating cancer becomes your number one priority and all you want to do is get moving on the process. But like baseball or cricket, the health care system moves at its own pace, which is never as fast as you would like. As I navigated the system, the refrain, "Come on! This is my life. Hurry up!" went through my head daily.

You will wait to get appointments. You will wait for insurance approvals. You will wait to get your records. Each wait is agonizing, but always be nice and be patient.

But—and here's where self-advocacy comes in—don't be too patient. Push, if needed. Here are a few tips to help you on your way.

The care team: How to pick and how to manage them

First, ask your primary care physician for a recommendation as to where to go to get your cancer treated. Then, go online and do your homework. This is where asking family and friends can come in handy, too. Also, read reviews.

Picking your care team may be the most important decision you will make in your cancer journey. The seriousness of picking the right care team *for you* cannot be understated. The work I did to find the right places for my care has paid big dividends. Moving from a small for-profit oncologists' office to larger medical facilities, either a dedicated cancer center or a facility with a special cancer department, was worth the effort.

You must find your cancer's experts. You don't take a Ferrari to a Chevy dealership. You are a Ferrari. When you think of where to go for care, also look for cancer centers with great reputations that treat a high volume of patients with your particular type of cancer. To find them, it will take research. You can find National Cancer Institute (NCI)-designated cancer treatment centers throughout the US via cancer.gov. As of 2022, sixty-four provide cancer care. But there are many other places in the US and around the world that also provide great cancer care. For example, in Canada, the Princess Margaret Cancer Centre. Other examples of very well regarded cancer centers include the Charité Comprehensive Cancer Center in Germany, SNU Cancer Hospital in South Korea, Peter MacCallum Cancer Centre in Australia, and Royal Marsden Hospital in the UK.

Some of the specialized cancer centers have affiliations with other medical facilities. For example, the MD Anderson Cancer Center partners with hospitals in many cities to provide cancer care using MD Anderson protocols and resources. Picking your care team is a personal decision, driven by many factors, including your ability to travel and insurance coverage. Just do the research and find what is best for you and your situation. The key here is that YOU decide where you go.

Like buying a car, you will want to check out different models and compare dealers. Do this for your cancer journey, too.

Benefits of high-volume cancer centers

Frequency of patients provides high-volume cancer centers with greater expertise. You want to go somewhere that has seen a LOT of patients with your type of cancer. These facilities should have specialists for your particular type of cancer. If not, find one that does.

Access to and even the development of a large number of clinical trials is a big advantage. The high-volume centers in the US have relationships with the NCI, as well as the pharmaceutical companies. Plus, with the volume of patients they see and the expertise they have, those big places will work to create clinical trials. For example, the trial I was in for my first lymphoma was developed by an MD Anderson doctor in conjunction with two pharmaceutical companies.

Access to the latest equipment is also an advantage. The high-volume cancer centers have the latest and greatest. The equipment piece extends to surgical equipment, radiation treatment—all of it.

The teams at the high-volume facilities may have developed surgical and care treatment protocols not commonly utilized by others.

Many will also deal with the rare cancers.

They understand the importance of speed in getting you in to see them. They will do everything to move it along for you. They can handle a lot of patients!

Picking your care team may be the most important decision you will make in your cancer journey.

Other benefits of high-volume cancer care facilities include:

- Having an easy-to-use online portal and app, which is great for scheduling, communicating, keeping records, and more.

- 24/7 availability while going through treatment.

- Broad insurance coverage, with a large number of health insurance companies. If your health insurance plan does not cover you at one—ask the health insurance provider for an exception and then ask the cancer center for help.

- Better service due to larger staff. Both my care teams treat me like a family member. Their attitude is great. Numerous times, I have been lost finding my way to an appointment. I remember one occasion where the cleaning person took the time to show me where to go. Top to bottom, the staff are trained to keep an eye on the patients.

- More treatment options for your cancer. Not just clinical trials, but experience and expertise with your particular type and sub-type.

- Coordinated treatments for patients like me, with more than one cancer, should that be necessary.

- A wide range of support services. They can assist with most issues you might have, including mental and emotional help, direction on financial support, travel support, housing support, nutritionists, physical therapists, and social workers.

- Satellite options for testing and meeting with doctors, enabling a patient to benefit from a smaller environment, perhaps closer to your home. For example, the Mayo Clinic campus in Jacksonville is super nice, but not large. It is like a very nice university campus with manicured lawns, ponds, and fountains. I can walk across the entire campus in fifteen minutes. When I had my lymphoma surgery there, the biopsy was sent to the much larger Mayo Clinic headquarters in Rochester, Minnesota. There, the team did the genetic analysis to determine my sub-type of lymphoma.

- Ability to attract some of the best of the best staff for cancer treatment.

After choosing your care team

Once you have picked your care team, it's time to meet with them to review results to date and next steps. During those appointments and all future appointments, listen intently and avoid any distractions. Here are some tips for meetings you have with your care team:

- Prepare for each meeting by doing your research. You must get an A+ on this test. Research your type of cancer in detail; try to understand the biology of your cancer and its treatment options.

- During appointments, listen, take notes, ask questions, build relationships. Dress well for these appointments, in business casual, as a sign of respect.

- After appointments, mail a handwritten thank-you note to those you met. I do this frequently—and am surprised how much they appreciate it. So, make a difference and do it!

- Always know the details of your case. Know your type of cancer, sub-type of cancer, timetable, symptoms, any history with it. When and where symptoms started. Medications you take. All of it. I have a two-page document that summarizes my health, including my cancer. This is the overview the doctors may need. I provide it to each new member of my care team during my first appointment with them.

- While it may not seem relevant, track non-cancer health issues, too. The fact that since I turned thirty, I have had my appendix, thyroid, tonsils, and multiple tumors removed, and had eye surgery, hemorrhoid treatment, and back surgery, might be relevant. It sure came in handy to the radiologist noting the absence of my appendix and thyroid in the first CT scan for my lymphoma diagnosis.

- Coordinate and communicate all health issues with all your doctors—both cancer and non-cancer. This YOU must coordinate. Ensure all your doctors know about your cancer, treatment, and any other health issues you are dealing with now or have dealt with in the past. For example, chemotherapy can damage the heart. Any past heart data should be shared across your cancer doctors, primary care physician, and cardiologist. This takes a lot of effort and a lot of organization. I had a crazy rash on my arm during my last round of chemo-therapy. I went to my local dermatologist, showed her, got the results, and then communicated those back to the Mayo Clinic. They noted it and kept an eye on it during my chemo visits. In fact, it prompted the surgical installation of my infusion port.

- Keep your health records available and organized. For example, as I write this, I am just back from the Mayo Clinic. The purpose of my trip was for the clinic to review my thyroid cancer history, to check to make sure it had not returned, and to review my thyroid medications to make sure they were correct. Clinic staff asked me to provide my thyroid surgery biopsy report, which was critical to understanding the sub-type of my thyroid cancer. First, I knew the answer. Second, I emailed them the biopsy report. It was from 2002 and I had it! It took me two minutes to find it. Why? I had provided my thyroid medical records to the MD Anderson Cancer Center in 2003 when I got a second opinion—and the biopsy report and other information was on my MD Anderson portal. Booyah!

- When meeting with your care team, ask them a lot of questions. Keep a list of questions—and ask away. They will be happy to answer them. They like educated patients. Review these questions with your appointment buddy (see Chapter 9) ahead of time. You don't want to miss any questions. To get in all the questions you need to ask, save the chitchat with the care team until after your questions are answered. Then, write down the answers and save them.

- Be open to changing teams, if needed. I switched to the Mayo Clinic for my lymphoma treatment because the cancer came back during the pandemic, and MD Anderson could not take me quickly due to COVID-19 protocols. Thankfully, it is only a four-hour drive from my home to the Mayo Clinic (Jacksonville campus). I have known cancer patients who switched care centers because of poor customer service or bedside manner. Some switch at the advice of their care team, after being told they need more specialized care.

- Always stay on top of current and future treatment options for your type of cancer. For example, I am talking with both my care teams already about treatment options for my impending fifth bout with lymphoma, so I am prepared when it comes back. Both are discussing different potential treatments. Both know the research that is being done and the testing that is happening with the next generation of treatments. The point is that you must know the options and discuss them with your care team(s).

- Manage the other areas of your life that will impact your healing. Reduce stress the best you can, eat a healthy diet, get enough sleep, stay hydrated, exercise if you are able.

- Advocate for yourself in regard to any emotional or mental health issues you may be having. Review these with your care team. Don't try to hide them. The care team will have resources, but if they do not have what you need, get some outside help.

- Communicate frequently with your cancer care team, not just when they ask you or expect you to communicate. The easiest way is to keep them updated through emails or the patient portal. They not only want to know, but need to know how you are doing. Call them if anything serious comes up. Issues will come up. Let them know immediately. When in doubt, call. You are NOT bothering them.

- Know in detail the medications you are being prescribed. Know the doses you are taking, and side effects you are experiencing, and track them. Then, tell your care team if you are having issues.

- Tell the team if you are drinking alcoholic beverages during treatment (even if just a beer a week) or using marijuana or any other drugs. They need to know.

- Try and have a great relationship with your health care insurance provider (I do, with Cigna via Healthgram, thanks, Stephanie J.). That relationship is very valuable.

- Take charge of lining up the support you need. Friends, family, therapists, nutritionists, personal trainers.

Above all, own it!

Stay organized

Leverage online resources. In many cases, you can request appointments and records online. My advice: When you get an appointment with a doctor, take the earliest date they offer. I always ask for the first available appointment. I also ask them to call me if anyone cancels, so that I can get in earlier. Why? Beating cancer is my number one priority.

Be super organized. I use the Notes app on my iPhone, which is synced to upload to the cloud so I can also access the notes on my laptop. I physically take notes with a pen and paper on calls or during appointments and then scan those using my iPhone and place them into Notes, then back them up using Microsoft's OneDrive. This way, I always have access to all the information I need.

Track who you call, when you call, the number you call, and the outcome of the phone call. Use whatever system works best for you—but stay organized! Even if you had a great memory before hearing the news, your memory won't be as sharp because of the challenge of balancing your new job of beating cancer with all of your other priorities, as well as the cancer fog from treatments.

6

NEXT STEPS OF THE JOURNEY

WITH YOUR care team in place, you will go through a medical process regarding the cancer. The goals of this process are to:

- Confirm that you have cancer.
- Identify the exact type of cancer.
- Determine how much the cancer has spread (called staging).

With this information, your care team will develop a treatment plan specifically for you.

For example, there are many different sub-types of lymphoma within the two most common lymphoma types. All this testing needs to happen to make sure the right type and sub-type of cancer is treated, whatever cancer you may have.

Screening and symptoms

Screening tests are conducted in order to catch cancer early, sometimes before you even have symptoms. These can include blood tests, biopsies, genetic testing, and imaging tests. Some are prescribed to you proactively. A mammogram, colonoscopy, and a Pap smear are examples of screening tests done regularly, depending on a patient's age and health. Medical advances are adding more diagnostic tools to the "catching cancer early" toolbox.

But screening tests can't catch everything, or not always in time. The process of getting into the Cancer Club often starts with you knowing something is not quite right with your body. You see it, you feel it, you sense it. Once you notice an issue, your first visit is usually with your primary care physician. The primary care physician prescribes tests and refers you to specialists (or your care team) for those tests.

Types of tests

Here are some standard cancer screening tests you can expect:

- Blood tests. These are a great way for the doctors to understand aspects of your cancer (e.g., prostate-specific antigen (PSA) tests for prostate cancer).

- Scans. The major types of cancer scans are: CT, computed tomography, or "cat" scans; MRIs, magnetic resonance imaging scans; and PET, positron emission tomography, or "pet" scans. You could get a combined CT (or cat)/PET scan. (A cat-pet scan. Funny!) Bone scans are completed using nuclear imaging to determine if cancer has spread into the bones.

- X-rays. These tend to be quick. You can sit, stand, or lie down. It all depends on the location of the area being X-rayed. (Fun fact: When Wilhelm Röntgen discovered electromagnetic radiation in 1895, he did not know the type of radiation, so called it an X-ray.)

- Internal or external ultrasounds. You may get instructions for the test, which you will need to follow. The great thing about these tests is that the technician is with you the whole time, moving the equipment over your body (external) or sometimes in it (internal). You can usually talk with the technician during the test. Some technicians will even allow you to watch the monitor as they work. If they offer this option, take it. It is so cool to see your insides.

- Bone marrow biopsy and aspiration tests. These are performed with a needle and are common with blood cancers. These tests take samples from inside your bone. It is called a bone marrow biopsy if the sample from the marrow is solid. It is called a bone marrow aspiration if the sample from the marrow is liquid.

What to expect from your test experience

For the CT, MRI, and PET scans, you will lie on a table about the width of your body. They are not wide—nor are they heated! This table is connected to a machine. The magical testing is done while you are in the hole of what looks like a giant donut. The rooms are kept cold to prevent the machines from overheating. Thankfully, staff will

Follow the preparation instructions **exactly.**

cover you with heated blankets (if they don't, ask for one!). Some scans can be quick, some take longer. My typical CT and PET scans last under thirty minutes, not including the preparation time at the testing location. My longest MRI was ninety minutes. For MRIs, you will be provided headphones. Those machines are quite noisy (it sounds like someone banging loudly on a drum—the sound of magnets working in the machine). The headphones dampen the noise a bit, allow you to listen to music, and give the staff the ability to communicate with you during the test.

When the technician says don't move, they mean it. Any movement could result in a blurry scan, requiring the technician to re-shoot that piece of the test. Sometimes a voice that sounds like Amazon's Alexa will ask you to hold your breath, with the purpose of avoiding any movement caused by breathing. Don't worry, she will tell you when to breathe again, too. Those hold-your-breath moments don't last very long.

It is common to drink "oral contrast" while at the testing center, to prep your body for a CT scan. The contrast is a dye that highlights specific areas being scanned. You may be asked if you are allergic to iodine. You drink it out of a big plastic cup (or two) over a prescribed period. Don't worry, just prior to the scan you will be asked if you need to empty your bladder. You may also get an injection of contrast, delivered remotely, while on the table for a scan. The IV needed for this contrast will have been inserted before you start the scan. This contrast quickly travels through your body through your circulatory system. It will feel like a hair dryer moving over your skin. The heat starts at the face and neck and moves its way down your body. This is the part I don't like—it makes you feel like you soiled yourself. No one gave me a heads-up about contrast on my first CT scan. I was 100 percent sure I had soiled myself during the scan. After the scan was over, I sat up, looked, and realized I had not. Booyah! Small victories.

With PET scans, your pre-test diet is super strict. You must remove sugars well in advance of the scan. Again, follow instructions exactly. Drink a soda before the test, eat a candy bar, a bagel—and the test is canceled. Period. No second chance is likely that day, due to scheduling challenges combined with the time needed for your body to clear that food out of your system. In addition, you will be asked to refrain from any strenuous physical activity starting twenty-four hours before the test.

Prior to the PET scan, you will receive a radioactive isotope, called a tracer. This will be injected through an IV before the test. At the Mayo Clinic, to keep the nurses safe from radiation, a robot administers the tracer. The nurse simply connects the machine to your IV. Once injected, you will be isolated for an hour or so, to let the isotopes move throughout your body. During this time, relaxation is super critical. No phone, no reading, no talking. Just listening to music on headphones or sleeping. I listen to "chill" songs on Spotify. The reason for the relaxation is simple. The scan is so sensitive, you need to minimize thinking, lest too many isotopes head to the brain. It is harder to relax than it sounds—but you can do it! The PET scan, to me, is the miracle test. It literally lights up the locations of the cancer, at the cellular level. I get them after the initial cancer diagnosis and then during follow-up testing post-cancer. My first PET scan was with my first lymphoma. On the scan, my body was lit up like a neon sign—the cancer had spread throughout my body. Even I could understand the image. That news was not good—but at least we knew the locations of the cancer. CT and MRI scans are also great at finding cancer, they are just used in different ways.

Drink a lot of water after your scans. For CT, PET, and MRI scans, you want to flush out all the stuff that was injected into you or that you drank. For PET scans, be careful around kids and pregnant women for about twelve hours. You are literally radioactive, so stay away from them to keep them safe. After sixty hours there should be no trace of the radiation in you.

Don't bother asking for an early read of the scans. Before you can get up from the table, with the machine off, the technician will review the images to make sure they got what they needed for the doctor. Even if you are anxious to know the results of the scan, don't ask the technician for results or how it looked. They can't and won't tell you. The images will be sent electronically to a radiologist so that they can read them. The results will be shared with you by your doctor—or will show up in your online portal. Trying to read your results from the online portal is like opening a big can of worms. I recommend just waiting to review the results with your care team. Despite twenty years of trying, I still understand little of what is in those reports. And don't look at the technician and try to guess your test results by interpreting their expression. They are like poker players. Don't bother trying to figure out what they have seen. You can't.

Don't be concerned about the radiation from imaging tests. There are risks for certain scans, but they are not high. The higher priority is the cancer, so don't stress about the radiation from tests.

Here are some tips to improve your scan, X-ray, or ultrasound process:

- Don't arrive early and expect to get the scan early. Some places will start on time. Some will always start late. But never early. It just makes the waiting room crowded if you arrive early. Arrive on time.

- Follow the preparation instructions exactly. They may ask you to fast, perform an enema, stay off certain meds, or not eat certain foods. These instructions help ensure the most accurate scan results. Study the instructions, even if you've had a similar scan before. The staff will ask—and if you have not followed the correct preparation procedures, they will move your scan to another time.

- Wear clothes with no wires or metal in them. I wear sweatpants, slip-off tennis shoes, and a short-sleeve athletic shirt so staff can easily access my arms for an IV. Some testing areas will require you to change into medical scrubs, while others will allow you to wear your own clothes. But your clothes cannot have metal in them (this includes underwire in bras).

- Leave all jewelry at home or in the hotel safe to avoid dropping or losing anything. Don't plan for your hospital or clinic to have a secure spot for valuables, though most will have a locker available.

- Through trial and error, I have learned how to relax while going through these tests. While on the table for a CT, MRI, or PET scan, I will meditate or use my imagination to pretend I am somewhere else other than on

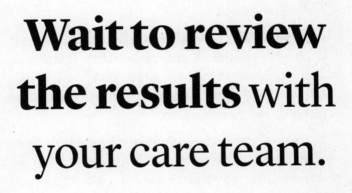

Wait to review the results with your care team.

a table, going in and out of a tube. I usually imagine I am on the beach, sitting in the sun, and listening to the waves. Use your mind to ensure you are relaxed and stay perfectly still.

- The staff will communicate with you during the test over speakers or via headphones. For safety reasons, the staff are behind glass in an adjoining room, with the exception of ultrasounds. Listen to what they say and feel free to ask a question during breaks that take place during the scan.

- Close your eyes during CT, PET, and MRI scans. There is a bright light shining onto you as the table you're on goes in and out of the tube, so you don't want to look into it. Closing your eyes can help with meditating, relaxing, and visualizing, too.

- Don't leave a PET scan and go to the airport to fly somewhere. Many airports have radiation detectors. It is a long shot, but after a PET scan you could set them off. Think about trying to explain that to airport security. If you are flying after a PET scan, bring documentation that indicates you have undergone a PET scan.

How to ace your biopsy

Biopsies are another way to confirm cancer and the specific type or sub-type of cancer. Biopsies are great, as they allow the doctors to conduct many tests on the tissue. A biopsy can happen a few different ways:

- A needle biopsy, to take out a piece of tissue from a tumor. These can be easy needle biopsies or complicated needle biopsies. The term *needle* can be a bit misleading. I was once awake for a needle biopsy on a tumor in my groin area. Those were some very big needles, with multiple tissue samples taken.

- A skin cancer biopsy, when a piece of the cancer is cut out and then sent to a lab.

- A surgical biopsy, treated like any surgery. You will be in a pre-operating room, be rolled to the surgical suite, and then given anesthesia. You will wake up in the recovery room with the biopsy complete. I have had surgical biopsies of my neck, throat, prostate, and groin area. Recovery from these surgeries varies. For these biopsies, follow the pre-operating instructions and the post-operating instructions. After a biopsy, stay hydrated, eat protein, rest, sleep, don't exercise. I have mixed emotions regarding the use of narcotics and discuss with the doctors pre- and post-surgery about whether I will need pain medication after the surgery. I almost always avoid taking the narcotics. Over-the-counter medications usually handle the pain. The reason I try to avoid narcotics is because of their side effects, including constipation, addiction, brain fog, and the inability to stay awake. Talk with your care team about it—but make your own decision regarding narcotics. The caveat here, though, is not to let the pain get out of control, as that can inhibit healing.

- Bone marrow biopsy/aspiration. As lymphoma is a blood cancer, this test is a common one for lymphoma patients. In this test, samples of bone marrow are taken using needles. The technician will go through the skin in the area around your hip, through the bone to the marrow inside the bone to pull out multiple samples of the marrow (where blood cells are made). Those samples will be placed on slides during the procedure and sent to a lab for analysis. You will be lying on your stomach on a table. I have always been wide awake for this test, but sometimes they are done with light sedation. You will get small injections of anesthesia in the test area. Once the marrow needle is inserted into your bone, there is no way to prevent bone pain unless you are sedated. This pain is very intense and unique. Inadvertent groaning, gasping, or crying is common during this portion of the test. Thankfully, the pain is short-lived, only when the needle is in the bone. The Mayo Clinic suggests the biopsy technician count down the amount of time that the needle will be in your bone. This way, you focus on the counting—and voila—the test is complete. This test takes under an hour, but the time the needles are in your bone is quite short. After the test, you will be bandaged up over the extraction sites. Outside of some soreness in that area for a day or two, you will feel A-OK after this test, though you may walk like you just got off a horse.

Staging your cancer

Staging is the process of identifying the size of your cancer and how much it has spread throughout your body. This provides a benchmark on how to best treat the cancer and how quickly to get moving. Staging is done on a scale of one through four. The lower the number, the less it has spread.

Along with staging, you will be provided a grade for your cancer—simply, what the cancer cells look like under a microscope compared with normal cells. The lower the grade, the better.

The staging and grading criteria vary by type of cancer. Let your medical team explain staging for your particular cancer and what it means. You can also look it up online, but don't spend too much time researching it. Lean on your care team.

For my first lymphoma, I was stage three, grade one, non-Hodgkin's follicular lymphoma. For my initial pros-tate cancer diagnosis, I was at stage two. I was also given a Gleason score, a specific numerical score for grading pros-tate cancer cells—again, the lower the better. The Gleason score is determined by adding up the two Gleason grades, which measure the appearance of cancer cells compared to non-cancer cells; together, they indicate the growth rate of the tumor (the overall Gleason score). So, I was a stage two, Gleason six (on a scale of six to ten).

Advances in genetic testing add another level of insight into a cancer. For example, the BRCA gene test (from a blood sample) identifies gene mutations that make patients more susceptible to breast cancer, prostate can-cer, ovarian cancer, and more. Genetic testing can also help identify the most effective type of treatment for your cancer.

7

THE BUSINESS OF CANCER

NO MATTER where in the world you live, there are certain business issues that you will need to handle as a cancer patient. It is unfair—but a reality—that you will need to deal with the business and the financial stress of cancer as well as the cancer itself. I cannot even guess how much cancer has cost my family financially over the past twenty years.

Being in the Cancer Club is expensive. There is no way around it. This won't change in the short term. So be ready for it. As a member of the club, you are already experiencing it.

Working

Having a full-time job while going through the cancer journey adds complexity to the journey and depends on your ability to continue work. Which in turn depends on the severity of your cancer and its treatment side effects. Many cancer patients, like me, have no choice but to work during treatment, as a result of financial and insurance needs.

For my thyroid cancer treatment and my first three lymphoma treatments, I continued to work full time. I would schedule my lymphoma treatments on a Friday, using a

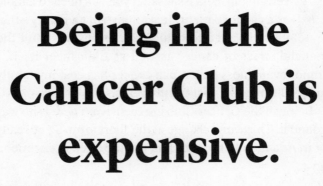

Being in the Cancer Club is expensive.
There is no way around it.

vacation day. I would fly to Houston after work on Thursday night. I would have my infusion on a Friday, fly back Saturday, recover a bit on Sunday and be back at the office on Monday morning. Most staff I worked with did not know I was going through treatment, though I did need to pull back on the number of hours I worked, due to fatigue. The side effects after treatment were largely manageable and because I did not lose my hair, I looked about the same, save for tiredness and steroid-induced weight gain. I used all sorts of tricks to hide my chemo brain, even going so far as to practice the math behind financial reports prior to meetings.

An accidental blessing happened with my fourth diagnosis of lymphoma. I had left my full-time job at the aquarium and started a marketing agency two weeks prior to receiving my diagnosis. But with my own marketing agency, and only one client, I could work as many hours a day as I felt I could handle, as long as I completed my tasks. My treatment side effects were quite challenging, so this modified work schedule provided a real benefit. I also worked from home, which was a huge advantage. I could not only hide side effects but handle them at home. I rested whenever I needed to rest. My time to remission beat expectations by three months. Not working full time and being able to rest, I am certain, helped me heal.

Other options

If I could wind back the clock, I would have worked less and rested more during all of my previous cancers. Perhaps I would have shifted to part-time work, taken a leave of absence, worked from home, used up my vacation time, or used disability insurance. I recommend this route if you can manage it financially. I have even known some patients who quit their jobs in order to focus on beating cancer. A benefit of working part time is that it can help you financially plus help take your mind off the cancer.

Travel costs

Travel costs can be a financial burden if you travel for care. Dr. Nathan Fowler, my doctor at MD Anderson Cancer Center in Houston and one of the world's greatest lymphoma oncologists, has seen this firsthand. One of his lymphoma patients, also from Florida, who was traveling to Houston often for treatment, told Dr. Fowler before he passed away that cancer had left him destitute. This gentleman left a wife and two kids with depleted resources. He had left his job to fight cancer, incurred the travel costs getting to and from treatment in Houston, and paid for the cost of staying in Houston during treatment.

In response to this story, Nathan and his mother, Kathleen Fowler, started the Halo House Foundation (halo housefoundation.org), which provides housing for adult blood cancer patients traveling to Texas Medical Center for treatment. Nathan knew that many of his patients were from out of town and needed a place to stay. His organization now provides fully furnished apartments to adult patients from outside of Houston. The Ronald McDonald House is an example of another amazing organization that provides accommodation support, but for sick kids.

Insurance

In the US, private health insurance can be quite expensive, with deductibles and co-pay portions in the tens of thousands of dollars per year. This can become a financial burden for many, if not most, patients using private insurance.

The business of cancer magnifies the importance of life insurance and disability insurance. Fortunately, I purchased life insurance before my first cancer, as I would not be able to purchase it now. If you have either life or disability insurance, make sure your coverage doesn't lapse and that you read the fine print. My private disability insurance has a wait period of 180 days, the same length as my cancer treatment, which brings with it reduced value. But if you are lucky enough to have disability insurance, look at that policy and consider using it. You can ask your employer, too, if they have a short-term disability policy.

The social workers at most cancer centers will have resources to help you identify ways to access financial support. Try to negotiate better rates or other benefits related to your cancer journey. I call this *using the cancer card*. At hotels, let them know when making your reservation that you are staying with them in order to receive cancer treatment. They might be able to provide you a better rate or more flexibility on checkout times. For airlines, work with your cancer center to try and get deals, if not on the flights, then on any changes to the flights. Some of the big cancer centers have deals or free tickets with the major airlines.

If you are in the US and your health insurance is insufficient for your cancer care needs, talk with your care team and ask for assistance or a payment plan for your medical expenses. In some cases, insurance won't approve tests requested by your care team. In this case, you will need to get help from your doctor to push the insurance company to approve it. A care team member talking directly with the insurance company usually gets it done. In some cases, you may still not get a test approved, and will have to decide if you are able pay for it yourself, out of pocket.

Lean on charities for help, too. There are many focused on specific types of cancer that provide financial and other support. For example, early in my battle, the Leukemia and Lymphoma Society was not only a source of information about my cancer, they also provided some funding for my travel. If needed, you can fundraise (using GoFundMe or a similar service) or ask someone to fundraise for you. This is common and often successful. Other cancer expenses include the cost of non-prescription medications and food for a revised and healthier diet. Even the cost of clothes when you gain or lose weight adds up. There is no way to avoid some of the expenses of cancer, so allow other people and organizations to support you.

Legal documents

This part is important for a couple of reasons. You want your wishes and desires known to others should you become unable to make your own decisions, or in the worst-case scenario, pass away. Outline your desires in legal documents. Make these important decisions while you are well so you or someone else does not need to handle them while you are sick and under enormous stress. As hard as

You can make your decisions easier for your family by **officially documenting them early in your cancer journey.**

it may be to handle these big questions, it is also the right thing to do; you can make your decisions easier for your family by officially documenting them early in your cancer journey.

This includes being prepared to make decisions about your health care easier and quicker. Many cancer centers will require documents to be completed prior to starting treatment. Common legal documents include a medical power of attorney, so that someone else can make medical decisions if you cannot make them, and a do-not-resuscitate document (or DNR) if that is your wish. A living will, which tells people the care you want if you cannot tell them; organ donation forms; and a will are also important, just in case.

My wife and I hired a lawyer who specializes in these types of documents. We had all of them completed when I started my journey. However, I only recently completed a "just in case" personal handwritten file which lays out additional non-legal details I want my family to know. I gave it to my wife, so she would have it—and hopefully not have to read it. For your "just in case" file, provide details about:

- How to access your phone.

- How to access your social media accounts (don't forget to change your settings so a legacy contact can handle them for you).

- Any financial issues that your family may not know about.

- What to do with your remains and the type of funeral you want.

- How you want your prized personal items distributed.

- Short notes to your family and other loved ones.

- Any other non-legal details you need others to know.

Having a "just in case" file for my family allows me to sleep better at night. I know that they will follow my wishes. I know, too, that I have made things easier for them. You should do the same.

You cannot avoid the business of cancer, so know the issues and manage them accordingly. My journey improved as I gained an understanding of the business of cancer. Cancer forced me to alter how our family spent our money, but the return on our investment has been priceless.

8

THE TREATMENT PLAN

YOU WON'T always know what lies ahead of you on your journey, and you won't be able to plan for all of it. But having a plan helps.

Plan development

Getting cancer today is better than getting it yesterday. Treatments are advancing rapidly and are fine-tuned for each individual based on your cancer and your situation. Many cancer centers use a team approach, looking at the data about the cancer and determining as a team the best treatment plan. Once they agree, they present that to you, the client.

When reviewing a treatment plan, you have to really be on your A game, organized and prepared. When MD Anderson presented my first lymphoma treatment plan to me, I turned it down because the treatment they recommended meant I would lose my hair. I was in sales and marketing at the time. Losing my hair would impact my job. As all good salespeople know, you must put the focus on the customer, not you. The team listened, took that as a challenge, and enrolled me in a clinical trial, developed

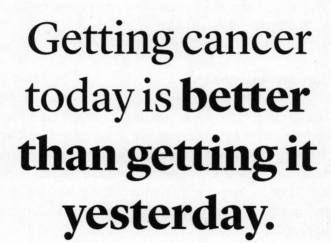

Getting cancer today is **better than getting it yesterday.**

by a doctor at MD Anderson and two pharmaceutical companies (Genentech and Bayer). In 2008, the word *immunotherapy* had not yet made it into the mainstream lexicon. I had never heard the word before. They explained it to me and told me if it did not work, we would go back to their initial plan. But the trial was worth a try and I would get to keep my hair—as well as avoid a litany of other side effects that came with the original treatment plan. I had accidently become part of history—an early benefactor of immunotherapy, which is now a common and effective way to treat cancer. By that time, I knew how to prepare, listen, challenge, and ask questions. Without those skills—I would have not been a part of history and would have been without my hair! Immunotherapy was used to help save me four times.

So do your homework, ask about your treatment plan, and understand its risks and side effects. Ask about clinical trials. The great places won't mind. They will listen to you. They want what is best for you.

Seek a second opinion

After you have been staged and have a treatment plan, and before you start treatment, go and get a second opinion. (The exception would be if the cancer is urgent and requires immediate treatment.) A second opinion may uncover a treatment plan that you feel is better. It will make you feel better, too, by getting someone else to weigh in on the initial plan and diagnosis. You are advocating for yourself! Cancer centers understand the importance of second opinions and do it as standard practice. I have found the high-volume cancer centers support second opinions going both directions—from them and to them. Most will move quickly to facilitate. Let your initial care team know you want to get a second opinion. Ask them for a recommendation on where to go to get a second opinion or find one on your own. Your care team will likely need to provide information and test results to wherever you go to get the second opinion, so don't keep it from them. With two opinions in hand, make your choice, and then lean into the care team you pick. Trust your judgment. You will make the right choice.

After your care team and treatment plan are finalized, you will schedule the treatments.

If you are given options, always take mornings over any other time. Treatments can be hard—better to get them done early while you are rested, if possible. Starting early in the day also provides some wiggle room should your starting time get delayed, or should the treatment take longer than expected, which happens often.

Travel tips

Many patients choose treatment centers close to where they live. I have always opted to have the treatment at the medical center of my care team, which I did not pick based on location. I picked MD Anderson in Houston and the Mayo Clinic in Jacksonville over a local option. I want *them* involved in every aspect of my care, including treatment. Thus, I once traveled to MD Anderson in Houston twenty-three times in one twenty-four-month period, and now travel to the Mayo Clinic in Jacksonville often.

If flying, try and pick an airline that flies direct to your destination, non-stop in both directions. If you have a long drive to get treatment and can fly, fly in for the first treatment in order to gauge how you feel for travel afterwards. A short flight can be preferrable to a long car drive. I am grateful to Southwest Airlines for accommodating my schedule on trips to and from Houston at no additional cost to me every time I needed to make a change.

Driving is ideal if you live close enough, as you have unlimited flexibility in case of any changes to appointments or how you feel. You will thank me for this tip—don't valet park at the medical center if it is offered, even if it is free (you will still owe the tip). It is a great service, but the wait time to get your car after treatment can be very long. The last thing you want to do when leaving a cancer center is wait. Your goal will be to get back to your hotel or home— and *rest*! Plus, if you are immunocompromised, you don't want a stranger in your car.

Bring extra clothes, toiletries, and medications with you. Sometimes, you will stay an extra night or two—so be ready.

Where to stay

If you are staying overnight, staying with family or friends is great, as long as they are healthy.

If you need to or decide to stay in a hotel, apartment, or vacation rental, consider the following:

- Location. Preferably walking distance to the treatment center or a place with shuttle service to the treatment center.

- Food options available nearby. You usually won't want to eat out. Simple, plain food is best. No matter how much you are craving a big, fancy meal—skip it. Many nights pre-treatment I will eat a grilled cheese sandwich with some soup.

- Duration of your stay. Airbnb, VRBO, and Whimstay vacation rentals are great for long-term stays.

- Flexible cancellations. It is hard to predict when your treatment schedule will change.

Treatment types

I am not a doctor, and thus cannot recommend any one treatment over another. Below is a list of some of the more common treatments you may encounter. Ultimately your treatment is up to you and your care team. Modern medicine has saved me five times and I believe in it. Innovative treatments may get me to my goal of living to age ninety-three.

- Chemotherapy (or chemo). You are given drugs in pill form or intravenously. Getting cancer drugs through an IV is called an infusion. For chemotherapy, the drugs kill the cancer cells and some non-cancerous cells as well. Chemotherapy has been around for a long time and has been very effective at treating certain cancers.

Each cancer has **a unique treatment protocol.**

Each cancer has a unique treatment protocol. The doctors will talk about treatment being administered in cycles. A cycle is treatment followed by a period of rest or recovery. But a cycle does not always mean a day. For example, for my latest lymphoma chemotherapy and immunotherapy, I had six cycles, which included fourteen days of treatment, spanning six months. My first cycle lasted three weeks and included four treatments. Then, one month off for rest, and then five more cycles, two days each back-to-back, with one month off after each two days of treatment or cycle.

- Immunotherapy. You are given drugs either in pill form or intravenously. Sometimes, for skin cancer, you're given a cream that helps your body kill the cancer. With the help of the drugs, the cancer cells are killed by healthy cells in the body. Immunotherapy is deservedly getting a lot of great press. It is a great way to treat many cancers.

- Radiation. This comes in three main forms: Through medications, beam radiation, or radiation seeds. Radiation is targeted to kill the cancer (for example, the radioactive iodine-131 pill I was provided for my thyroid cancer). Beam radiation, or radiotherapy, is where a beam is directed at the cancer and kills it. In some cases, like with prostate cancer, radiation "seeds" will be implanted directly into the prostate and onto the cancer.

- Hormone therapy. Hormones are given to slow or stop the growth of cancers like breast and prostate cancer.

- Stem cell transplants. Blood-forming stem cells that have been killed by chemotherapy or radiation treatment are replaced with modified stem cells intravenously. The source of these healthy stem cells will be your own stem cells or someone else's that match.

- Targeted therapy. There are wide-ranging treatment options that target cancer cells with proteins or enzymes to block them from growing. This is also a form of chemotherapy, but unlike chemotherapy, the goal is not to kill non-cancer cells. You could argue some immunotherapies are also targeted therapies.

- Surgery. Some cancers can be removed completely with surgery. However, other treatments often follow the surgery to prevent the spread of cancer.

- "Watch and wait" or "active surveillance." We are following this plan currently with my prostate cancer. Blood tests, biopsies, and scans will be scheduled—but in this case, the approach is to wait, test, and only start treatment if the cancer grows.

Port or no port?

A port, or an implanted infusion/chemo port, is surgically inserted in your body with the intent to easily and quickly get medications into your body. Ports are commonly installed in the right chest, below the collarbone. They are round and not very large, and connect to a vein near the heart. They sit just under the skin, so are visible when wearing a tight shirt or with no shirt on. They are high tech, and made of a comfortable material. IV needles are inserted into the port, which closes back up once the IV needles are removed.

I did not have a port installed for my first three lymphoma immunotherapy infusion treatments and started with my fourth treatment regimen, which included immunotherapy plus chemotherapy, without one. However, after a few treatments, it became clear to my doctor that I needed a port installed. My arms and hands were swelling, and my skin was itchy and splotchy. Skin issues, vein issues, and swelling are common side effects when chemotherapy is delivered through the hands and arms. These symptoms can be alleviated with the installation of a port. The infusion staff like ports, too, for the consistency in administering medications and the fact that the port eliminates the need to find a good vein to take the needle.

The surgery to install the port was under an hour, and completed in the surgical suite of a hospital. I was under general anesthesia, thus asleep for it. Some patients have them installed only with local anesthesia.

The surgery to remove the port after treatment is not very physically painful. As I came out of the dressing room, after changing into surgical scrubs before the port removal surgery, a nurse observed me fumbling trying to open the locker where I was to put my clothes. She stopped and asked me how I was doing. I told her I was very anxious and scared about the surgery. She then suggested I take and then brought me an anti-anxiety pill. It made a huge difference for me. I was quite relaxed and awake as the doctor simply cut open the area (they had injected localized pain medications) where the port was installed and pulled it out. I walked out of the surgical suite after they cleaned me up and glued the incision shut. The doctor even showed me my port after it was removed from my body, after I asked to see it. The scar from it is now barely even visible.

Ports can stay in for years, but they do need to be flushed every four weeks. I had mine surgically removed as soon as I could, with my doctor's approval, after chemotherapy. I had it removed not because it bothered me physically, but because it reminded me of my cancer. Also, I did not want to worry about getting it flushed regularly.

Another option for administering medication is a peripherally inserted central catheter (or PICC line), which does not require surgery to install. Your care team will recommend the best option for you.

Length of the treatment plan

The length of the treatment plan depends on your cancer and type of treatment. My shortest treatment plan lasted three months. My longest treatment plan lasted six months, but many patients have much longer treatment plans. One year or more is not uncommon. Upon completion of your treatment plan, you will need time to recover, and recovery can take months.

9

THE BUDDY SYSTEM

CANCER PATIENTS need a buddy system for the cancer journey, in particular for appointments and treatments. Buddies are important in so many ways to the patient. I could not have successfully managed my journey on my own.

My buddy has been my wife, Kim. Countless times she has asked a great question of the care team, called them to let them know of a health issue during my infusions, walked me to the bathroom, changed a bandage, and even wheeled me in a wheelchair to the car. She has been my eyes and ears. Her role in the journey cannot be underestimated. There are no words that can communicate how much I appreciate her help as my buddy over the past twenty years.

Cancer is physically and emotionally challenging for Kim, too. It is hard to watch those you love suffer. Kim has witnessed a lot, with little ability to make me feel better other than to smile, say kind words, and hold my hand. When I am going through infusions, although we talk very little, we communicate often with our eyes and even by shaking our heads.

This is called the *buddy system*. The beauty of the buddy system is that the role of the buddy does not always need to be filled by the same person. If you are married or in a close relationship, your spouse or partner is an obvious buddy, but sometimes, they may have work or other commitments which require you to find another buddy. Or maybe your spouse or partner's health (physical, emotional, or mental) is not strong enough to provide the support you need at that time. If you are single, friends are great at being buddies! The good news is that your close friends will almost always ask if they can help you during your cancer journey. If you need them, ask them, and they will help. Saying yes to their offers of help is good not only for you, but for them. They will feel like they are a part of your team!

If no one can come with you to an appointment, ask your care team for some support. Most cancer centers have a great group of volunteers who would happily help you any way that they can.

However, while you can have many buddies during your journey, I strongly recommend only one at a time go with you to your appointments. More than one buddy makes it challenging for the care team to know who to communicate with if you cannot communicate. Plus, it brings an additional element of risk regarding bringing an illness into a care facility. Many care centers limit the patient to one buddy.

The job of being a buddy is a big responsibility. It must be taken seriously. A buddy will have to be prepared and do a lot of homework. Your buddy might ask a question or notice a health issue that could save your life.

Buddy requirements

Your buddy must be:

- Healthy when with you and, in particular, at your appointments. You can't risk them getting you or other patients sick.

- Emotionally strong.

- Well-spoken and organized.

- A good listener.

- An adult. In many cases, children are not even allowed to be with you during appointments or treatments.

You will need a buddy with you at your appointments to listen to the care team and to take notes. As a patient, stress and medications can make it difficult for you to comprehend what your care team tells you. Review with the buddy the goal of the meeting, and go through meeting notes in advance.

A buddy must accompany you to scans where you may be a bit off, physically or mentally, coming out of them. Buddies cannot go into a scan with you but are there when you leave. For me, the scans where I need a buddy included scans where I had fasted in preparation. I am thin, so fasting makes me a little light-headed. You also need a buddy for tests like bone marrow tests, which physically hurt, and for any scans which require sedation.

You need a buddy with you for infusion treatments. There is real risk to the patient during these treatments, so your buddy not only needs to be with you, but needs to be paying attention to you, as well. All the time! From reminding you to stay hydrated, to getting you food, to keeping you from falling on your way to the bathroom, to calling the nurse if you start to have a bad reaction, buddies are important. My wife handles my phone calls and texts during infusions, as well. During the pandemic, some cancer centers did not allow buddies; instead, the staff kept a vigilant eye on the patients.

The buddy will need to be prepared, like you. They must know about the doctor, the medical records, the medications you are taking, as well as the ones being administered to you. They should prepare a list of questions in advance of appointments. Even to the point of having a one-page summary of medical issues. So, the job of the patient is to educate the buddy on all of these issues.

The buddy system does not just work while you are with your care team, it also works at home. For the first two or three days after an infusion, even though you may sleep a lot, it is super important to have a buddy. This does not mean the buddy has to be with you 24/7, but that they can be available, if needed. I have needed my wife to call the doctor when something is wrong, and she has reminded me to take medications. My wife has kept people away when I am resting. She pre-screens all visitors who want to see me to ensure they are healthy. She makes sure I eat, including the best foods for my side effects.

Emotional support

The buddy is also helpful for emotional support. Choose someone who can listen and help you through it. However, the buddy is not meant to be your therapist or support

The beauty of the buddy system is that **the role of the buddy does not always need to be filled by the same person.**

group. If you need mental or emotional support, get help from a therapist or a support group. It is OK to lean on your buddy for some support, but leaning on them too much is not healthy for them.

Pets

. . . . . .

My sweet Cavalier King Charles Spaniel, Pippa, is a great buddy, too. Pets are terrific for cancer patients. Petting her, walking her when I can, having her sleep next to me, is therapeutic. Her excitement when I get home from the doctor makes me feel great, too. She is by my side often, and I love it. I jokingly call her my therapy dog—but it is not a joke. I highly recommend, if you are able, to have a pet during your cancer journey. While this buddy won't go to your appointments, pets are great for your heart and soul when you are home!

10

ACE YOUR TREATMENT

TOOK MY work computer to my first infusion thinking I would be able to get some work done, and maybe even make phone calls. I was clueless and learned quickly to clear my calendar on treatment days. Not just the first treatment day, but all of them.

You will be in no condition physically, mentally, or emotionally for anything other than getting the treatment. Focus on yourself. No one else. These are days when it is OK to be selfish.

Do not plan to make any big life decisions while you are undergoing treatment. Changing jobs, buying cars, making travel plans, and making other big spending or investment decisions... Leave those big decisions for a later time.

It is sign of strength to ask for mental health help. Many cancer patients ask for it; most of us need it. This is a great time to line up those resources.

Your buddy will need something to do while waiting with you, so remind them to bring books, headphones, phone chargers and spare batteries, a computer, snacks, water, and a sweatshirt or sweater. Have them bring something to take notes with if needed. And money, if necessary, for parking or food.

Anatomy of an infusion treatment
. . . .

Infusions can include chemotherapy and immunotherapy. The treatment can be quick or take hours. In some cases, you may be hospitalized for days, or, in many cases, be in and out of the infusion center on the same day. Note: the first treatment takes the longest for a lot of reasons, including giving you the meds at a slower pace to gauge how your body handles them. The staff can estimate the time you will be there. Just ask. But the infusion process can be a bit challenging to predict, as each person has a different reaction to the medications.

For most infusions, the process works like this:

- Prior to the infusion, you will have a blood test. They are checking the heart, kidneys, liver, white blood cell counts, red blood cell counts, and more. The goal is to green-light the patient for that treatment or cycle.

- Prior to the infusion you will meet with a member of the care team. They will take your blood pressure, your temperature, your weight, your heart rate, and review the data from the blood test. They will ask you how you are doing, probe any side effects, answer questions about the infusion, change pre-meds as needed, and prescribe medications for managing side effects. They will listen and probe to determine how you are doing mentally and emotionally. If there are issues, they will work to get you support. If you are having side effects or have any questions, have those in writing—and make sure you get them answered.

- During the infusion, you may be in a room with others or may have a private room for the treatment. All of my treatments have been in a private room. My cancer is of the immune system so keeping me away from others is critical.

- You will sit in a comfy chair or recliner or lie in a bed, depending on the facility and the treatment.

- The infusion staff will check your details and then review with you what medications you will be given. They, too, will ask about any side effects, and, if needed, reach back out to the care team with any questions.

- Before the cancer drugs are given, you will likely be given pre-meds to help prevent side effects.

- You may experience a negative reaction to the infusion. This is when your body's immune system responds to a drug you are getting. Reactions can happen with chemotherapy, immunotherapy, and targeted therapy. The key here is to ask about the possibility of an infusion reaction before you start your treatment or research it online. Ask what a reaction could be like. In many cases, the care team won't tell you unless you ask, as reactions are hard to predict for every patient. Don't be blindsided, like I was the first time I had a reaction. You could experience itchy skin, itchy scalp, hives, shortness of breath, a racing heart, chest pain, fever, chills, nausea, or more. Infusion reactions are common and always hard. Most can be managed effectively with a protocol already determined for you in case a reaction happens. But, as you will see from my personal experience, infusion reactions can be life threatening.

Ask about the possibility of an infusion reaction

before you start your treatment or research it online.

Risk of infusion reaction

In May 2008, during my first treatment for lymphoma, with no warning, I had a serious and life-threatening reaction to the immunotherapy drug that was being administered by a computerized intravenous machine. One hour into my first treatment, my wife had just left my private treatment room at MD Anderson to call our family to tell them all was going well. Unfortunately, the moment she left my room, the train came off the tracks. I went into anaphylaxis. Alarms went off and the nurse saw what was happening and immediately called for help, and then gave me a shot directly into my IV where it entered my body. Speed was key. They practice for moments like this and the nurse reacted perfectly. By then, I was already struggling to breathe, my eyes had largely swelled shut, my chest was tight, my heart rate was through the roof. I was in shock. It was like being allergic to bees and getting stung by a thousand at one time—but not knowing you are allergic to bees. It was just minutes, but it felt like forever. Plus, I had literally no idea this type of reaction was possible, as I had not asked nor done any research. None. Ignorance was not bliss.

At the time of my reaction, my wife happened to be outside of the hospital in order to get a good cell signal. By the time she came back to my infusion room, I was sedated, the room was dark, and the infusion IV machine was turned off. When she walked into the room, all I could do was sob. I had just suffered more than I had ever suffered before. At the moment of the infusion reaction, my life had been at risk, not just from the cancer, but from the treatment. I was thankful for the team that stabilized me, but I never looked at cancer the same way after. From that day on, the gravity of cancer and the seriousness of cancer treatment has never left my soul.

If you have a reaction, your cancer medication will likely be stopped while they address the side effects and work to control them, which can take a while. A reaction will lengthen your treatment time, as once the cancer drugs are started back up, they will slow the pace of administering them to allow your body more time to adjust. Once you have had a reaction, the care team will do everything possible to prevent it from happening again during future infusions. They do this with pre-meds. While you are in the treatment, tell your buddy and alert the staff if you feel itchy, your skin starts getting splotchy, you have a hard time breathing, or your heart rate goes up. Don't wait to tell someone. Pull the cord, push the button, or just yell for help. The moment you feel like something is wrong—tell them. It is an emergency.

Helpful treatment tips for infusions

- Don't eat a big meal before any infusion. A light meal is easier on the stomach.

- Do bring a bottle or two of water to drink during the treatment. Staying hydrated is key.

- Wear comfortable clothes. Sweatpants. Short-sleeve shirt. Zip-up sweatshirt. Slip-on shoes, with a rubber sole. You may be wobbly and don't want to slip when going to the bathroom.

- Wear warm socks.

- Bring a ski cap. Your head will get cold.

- Bring a baseball cap to keep light out of your eyes.

- Bring noise-canceling headphones. They'll drown out noise and allow for listening to music, podcasts, or audiobooks.

- Bring either a laptop, tablet, or cell phone so that you can watch movies if you are awake. Don't bother bringing books; it is hard to read them. If you want to read, magazines are better. Forget trying to work. Emails. Phone calls. Don't do it. Many infusion areas have TVs you can watch.

- The care team may provide you with blankets. If not, bring your own.

- Bring your cell phone charger, and extra batteries for headphones, if needed.

- Bring some snacks, in case you are hungry.

- Bring some mints or Life Savers in case you get a bad taste in your mouth from the meds.

- Bring sunglasses in case you cannot adjust the lights and want to keep light out of your eyes.

- Bring hand sanitizer and use it often.

- Bring lip balm for dry lips. Remember, those rooms are cold. This will keep your lips moist.

- Wear a surgical mask, if needed. Even post-pandemic, this is a great idea.

- Bring antibiotic cream to place on any cuts and make sure any cuts you have coming into the treatment have a bandage over them. The care team will likely ask about and look for any cuts before you start treatment.

Give your care team some grace if they are not as attentive as you desire. Some days, they have their hands full with other patients. The infusion center has a screen somewhere with your name on it and your status. One status is that there are no issues. Another status is often called Code Red, for a patient with an infusion reaction. Sometimes, there will be a Code Blue, for a heart issue or heart attack. The care team has an emergency plan for the Code Blues—a crash cart is already nearby, a team is trained to handle the patient, and an easy exit is already designated to get the patient to the cardiac care unit of a hospital. The more Reds and Blues, the busier the staff will be that day. The only time I ever had an issue with getting the highest level of attention was a day with a lot of Reds and, unfortunately, a Blue.

Stay safe, meaning DON'T GET SICK!

Your ability to fight illness is diminished, plus your cancer treatment will likely be slowed or stopped while you recover from an illness. It is the non-cancer illnesses that kill many going through the cancer battle. A cold, the flu, COVID-19—all become serious and potentially deadly to a cancer patient. A good friend, also a blood cancer patient, was beating his cancer, but unfortunately lost his life to

Each day, wake up and
remind yourself that
**your number one goal
is to beat cancer.**

COVID-19. When this happened, I ramped up my "stay safe" efforts even more.

I was diagnosed with cancers number five and six during the middle of the COVID-19 pandemic. In addition to having to switch care teams, COVID-19 emphasized the importance of not getting sick during treatment. Getting sick with COVID-19 during and after my treatments, based upon the survival data for blood cancer patients getting my treatment, would have meant increasing my chance of dying dramatically. In fact, as I edit this chapter, I am nine months post-chemotherapy, have had three COVID-19 vaccines, and still have no COVID-19 antibodies. My world is thus very small, as I need to be very, very careful.

Requiring masks when in cars with others, not seeing people if they are sick, and ensuring the family members and friends you see are vaccinated against COVID-19 and the flu, are all great at reducing your chances of getting sick. I know I will wear a mask into a doctor's office or hospital—forever.

Some tips to stay healthy:

- Wear masks around people inside. If anyone bothers you about it—just tell them you are immunocompromised.

- Avoid activities that are high risk. For example, I had to quit serving meals at a local homeless shelter. I attend church online. I avoid indoor crowds.

- When leaving appointments or treatment centers, go home or to wherever you are staying, leave your shoes at the door, take a shower, and wash your clothes.

- Prior to the start of treatment, with your doctor's insight and approval, get any vaccinations that will be helpful, as a vaccine may not work if received during chemo-therapy. Pre-chemo in 2020, per my doctor's direction, I received the flu vaccination. Ensure any vaccines you get are not "live" vaccines. Live vaccines can lead to serious illness in a cancer patient.

- Install an antibacterial and antiviral air purification system in your home, if you can afford it. We installed the Reme Halo system in our home—and it works. Hospitals use it, too.

- Monitor and log your temperature daily. If your temperature goes up, let your care team know. If it gets over 103.5 degrees Fahrenheit, head straight to the hospital. Make sure you have a plan as to which hospital you will visit if you get sick.

- Monitor your oxygen level daily using a finger pulse oximeter. They are inexpensive and a great way to determine if you may be developing a lung issue. Generally, any number below 95 percent is a red flag and warrants an immediate call to your care team.

- If you have blood pressure issues, monitor them, too.

- Wash your hands frequently, particularly before eating anything.

- Be careful where you eat. You do NOT want to get a stomach bug. In particular, don't eat from street vendors. Also, don't eat salads when out at restaurants. The lettuce could be contaminated. Avoid sushi, too. If something does not taste right or look right, don't eat it. It is not worth the risk.

- Be careful around your nose. Only scratch it with a tissue. Germs are on your fingers. Same goes for rubbing your eyes.

- Too much strenuous exercise can damage your immune system. Get your doctor's approval first. Light exercise can be good for you, so try to walk each day. The point of walking is to help your lungs. It is also great for mental health and dealing with the emotions of cancer.

- Eat a healthy diet.

- Be diligent about getting enough sleep. Take naps when you are tired.

- At least once a day, do some deep breathing. Breathe in through your nose counting to five. Hold it for five seconds and then breathe out slowly through your mouth. Repeat this five times. It will help you in many ways.

- Ensure you have alone time. Meditation is great.

- Dig into hobbies you enjoy.

- Binge-watch some shows.

- Help others. Helping others has been my secret sauce. This includes writing this book during my treatment, and talking with friends who are on their own cancer journey.

- Each day, wake up and remind yourself that your number one goal is to beat cancer. That will keep you focused.

Unfortunately, side effects are a part of many cancer treatments, not only infusions. The next chapter will help you be ready for them and manage them.

11

MANAGING
SIDE EFFECTS

THERE IS no way to sugarcoat it. Cancer treatment is tough. Not just physically, but mentally and emotionally. The day before a treatment I get pensive and moody—a bit more uptight, at times cranky. My family knows I just want to be alone. That's because the seriousness of the journey comes into focus, the fact that I am playing for keeps.

Side effects are also when the real physical suffering can start. This chapter will help lay out what to expect physically when going through treatment. The goal here is to not make you fearful, but to make you aware of the possible side effects so you can be prepared for them and manage them. Each patient reacts to medications in a different way. So, thankfully, don't expect to have all of these side effects. Almost all patients, though, do experience some side effects.

Prior to treatment, ask your care team about possible side effects from your medications. Not just the cancer-killing meds, but also the pre-medications and the meds helping mitigate side effects. You don't want any surprises. The care team, in general, does not have a lot of time to review these with you—so study them on your own, too.

Ask your care team, pre-treatment:

- What pre-meds am I going to get? Can you please take me through their potential side effects?

- What cancer meds am I going to get? Can you please take me through their potential side effects?

I know it sounds like a lot, but you'll be thankful for the extra information later. Go to the websites of the companies making the cancer drugs you will receive and review their research, too. Know who makes the medications and the side effects.

What side effects can you expect from your treatment?

It is difficult to know which medication is giving you which side effect, and you will receive a mix of medications—some oral, some intravenous, some injected. The side effects from the meds are all jumbled together, meaning it is hard to know which drug is giving you which effect.

Here are some common pre-meds and their side effects:

- Tylenol is a drug many are provided before each treatment. Most patients don't have side effects with it, but possible ones include headache, dizziness, sleepiness, and an upset stomach.

- Zofran and Pepcid are commonly given anti-nausea meds. They may make you constipated but they will prevent nausea.

- Benadryl, to manage allergic reactions, is commonly given prior to chemotherapy and immunotherapy. You may be sleepy. Your words may be slurred. Thinking becomes a real challenge. Your buddy becomes more important, here. You may have coordination issues, so get help walking to the bathroom. I learned this the hard way and tripped and cut my leg during a treatment. Dry mouth is also common.

- Dexamethasone (Dex), Solucortef, and prednisone. These are steroids and protect against infusion reactions. Dex is also used to fight my cancer. Side effects include difficulty sleeping for a few nights after getting them, and mood swings. I get large doses of both Dex and Solucortef. They make me very irritable. I try but cannot control it. Just ask my wife!

- Omeprazole, another common pre-med that reduces acid in the stomach, is given to reduce heartburn and indigestion. Common side effects include stomach pain and a headache.

- Side effects from cancer treatment are cumulative. The longer you are in treatment, the more pronounced the side effects become. It gets harder and harder as you go.

Always track your side effects, every day.

Aside from the side effects of the pre-meds, treatment (in particular chemotherapy, immunotherapy, and radiation) can have some challenging side effects. Some of the common ones include:

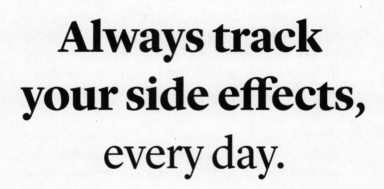

Always track your side effects,
every day.

- Chemo brain. It is real for some, but not all patients. Combine all the pre-meds plus the cancer meds with the stress and fatigue and no wonder it is hard to think. I felt about 15 percent off my pre-treatment ability to think. I was forgetting things, slower to understand things. Finding it harder to do math. Be aware, there is not much you can do for chemo brain other than compensate for it. For example, I have my wife remind me of the names of our friends before we see them. Make sure those around you know of your chemo brain and they can help, too.

- Chemo belly. This is simply the swelling of the belly due to weight gain, which can result from steroids and/or lack of exercise. I gained almost ten pounds during my last set of chemo treatments, all of it in the belly. Dammit! You will just have to wait it out. It will likely diminish on its own after treatment, as the medications wear off and you get more active.

- Fatigue. Your red blood cell counts may be low, so any exertion can make you out of breath. I was out of breath just going up the stairs, and once fell down the stairs because I was fatigued and wobbly. We then covered the stairs with anti-slip cloth. Expect fatigue, and sleep when tired. After treatments, I would spend days napping. Then, two naps a day. Then, one. Then, booyah, no naps about four months after my last treatment! My dog, Pippa, loved snuggling with me during all of them.

- Nausea. Super common. Stay on top of it. Don't let the nausea get out of control. Take the meds they prescribe.

You do not want to vomit, if at all possible, as you don't want to lose the nutrition. The challenge is that these anti-nausea meds can cause constipation. Big time. So, drink a LOT of water. If your care team approves, use medications and/or laxatives to help with constipation. Eat more high-fiber foods, if you can. You want to avoid an anal tear, also known as an anal fissure, which is caused by constipation and hard stools. I learned this lesson the hard way.

- Diarrhea can happen, too, and is common. Again, ask your care team immediately, if it happens, for medications to help control it.

- Reduced appetite.

- Infections. During chemo you are more prone to infections, even with the smallest cut. If you cut yourself, make sure to clean the wound frequently and even use an antibiotic cream. If you shave—use an electric razor to minimize the risk of cutting yourself. Be super careful in the kitchen. In fact, be super careful period not to cut yourself.

- Skin issues. Mouth sores are common. Your skin can get itchy, dry, and splotchy. I used a lot of lotion, and even dandruff shampoo for my head, to help deal with my skin issues. I used medications prescribed by the care team for the more challenging of them. These side effects can last for a while after the chemo treatments. Be careful not to get sunburned.

- Nail growth can slow way down.

- Blood pressure changes. Keep an eye on it with a home blood pressure kit.

- Heart rate changes and damage to your heart. I wear a watch that tracks my heart rate.

- Colds and coughs are common during treatment. Ask your care team which medications to take for these issues.

- Sense of taste and smell can change. In an odd surprise, during my last chemo treatments, my senses of smell and taste were enhanced. I even called the plumbers to fix a smell in my house. Two plumbers came to the same conclusion. They could not smell anything, but I could. The smell made me nauseated. They used a solution in the drains to get rid of what only I could smell. It worked. But for many, taste and smell become diminished. Over time, post-treatment, your senses get back to normal.

- Neuropathy. Numbness, tingling, weakness, or pain in your extremities (generally, feet or hands). Get in touch with your care team immediately if you have this issue.

- Loss of hair and a bald head. This is a common and expected part of going through chemotherapy. But losing your hair is not always a side effect of treatment. Your doctor can tell you if it is possible or likely you will lose your hair, based on the treatment you are getting. This way, you can prepare for it, if, indeed, it is likely you will lose all of your hair (on your head and elsewhere on your body).

The process of losing your hair can start as early as the first week after your first chemo, but for many it starts a little later. Many patients who know they are going to lose their hair make an event out of it, have a party, and shave their head. They use the occasion to get others to support them in their journey. Genius. During chemo, when hair starts to fall out, it comes out in clumps, in handfuls. All of a sudden. It is a jarring and very emotional moment for a cancer patient. So shaving your head before this happens or when it starts to happen makes sense. This way, YOU control the hair on your head coming off. If I were to shave my head, I would do it privately, as I know I would cry a lot. Many hair salons have a program for shaving off the hair of cancer patients. Some patients look great bald and stay bald. They wear their baldness proudly. Some patients try anything to keep the hair on their head, and there are products which can help. Cooling caps (e.g., DigniCap) keep your scalp cold during treatments and can (but are not guaranteed to) reduce hair loss. The large cancer centers will offer cooling caps as a treatment option. Ask your care team about it, if hair loss is a potential side effect and you want to minimize it. There are also stores that cater to providing wigs to cancer patients. I had a wig store lined up (thanks, Sarah Potts!) and ready to go in case all of my hair fell out. If you do lose your hair, remember to always have scarfs, hats, and ski caps available to help keep your head warm. You can choose colorful scarfs and hats to add some personality. Post-treatment, when your hair comes back (generally three to six months after your last treatment), your hair may come back differently. Maybe even soft and/or curly! In some cases, it will even come back a different color! My thinned hair grew back thicker.

Many patients who know they are going to lose their hair **make an event out of it, have a party, and shave their head.**

Diet to help with side effects

When you're too nauseous to eat, make sure you stay hydrated. Drink water and green tea with no sugar. It is great with ginger! Eat small meals more frequently, versus three big meals. Only take vitamins and other supplements upon approval of your care team. Some of them may impact the treatment effectiveness and can cause side effects.

Avoid entirely or reduce consumption of the following:

- Red meat
- Fried food
- Alcohol
- Salt
- Processed sugar
- Caffeine
- Dairy

Medical marijuana and cannabinoid drug use for side effects

The use of medical marijuana or cannabinoid drugs by cancer patients is a complex issue. Legality, availability, effectiveness, side effects, and quality vary greatly depending on where you live. My care team asked me not to use medical marijuana, as they did not know if and how it could impact the cancer-killing medications. I did not use it. However, it is used effectively by some cancer patients to help manage pain, nausea, and anxiety. If you are going to use medical marijuana, your care team will need to know details about how you are consuming it, how much, and the quality of what you are using. In many cases, they will need to prescribe it. In the US, there are some cannabinoid drugs approved for medical use. Your care team will recommend them, if needed.

12

EXPECT THE UNEXPECTED

LIVE IN a hurricane-prone area. I know what unexpected things to expect when a hurricane heads our way. I am prepared for it in many ways. When it comes, this preparation allows me to handle it better. This chapter will help you do the same, for cancer.

Cancer has a way of throwing you curveballs. Unexpected things will happen, so be mentally ready for the unexpected.

I thought that once I was diagnosed, had picked the care team, and had signed off on a treatment plan, my cancer journey would become more predictable. That it would be linear. I was wrong.

It is a zig-zag journey. You may get to the destination (beating cancer!), just possibly not on time and not via the route you expected to take. The care team will be cautious about sharing what "might" happen to you, as each patient is different and the unexpected can take many shapes and sizes. Some of the unexpected things that could happen during your treatment include the following:

Organs are impacted

The pre-meds, immunotherapy, radiation therapy, surgery, chemotherapy, and other treatments can have quite an impact on your body, unrelated to killing the cancer. You will be getting frequent blood tests with the specific purpose of identifying issues as they crop up and need to be managed. Your liver, heart, and kidneys will be reviewed, as will other areas of the body. If there are concerns with major organs resulting from your treatment, it will be paused and re-evaluated. Or it might be paused and restarted, if the danger diminishes. There is a lot of information available on how chemotherapy in particular can damage organs. Your care team knows this and will monitor you accordingly. Just this week, as I write this section, after chemotherapy, I was diagnosed with a new heart murmur.

Low white blood cell, red blood cell, and platelet counts

White blood cell, red blood cell, and platelet counts are reduced following chemotherapy, immunotherapy, and radiation therapy. Damage to your immune system is tracked with white blood cell counts. A reduction in red blood cells can cause fatigue and make it hard for you to catch your breath. A reduction in platelets can cause bleeding or make it hard to stop bleeding. Tracking this cell data can impact or change your treatment, force modified behavior, or provide information to the care team so they can prescribe medications to help resolve some of these issues. This data can also provide the care team insight on how the treatment is working.

Antibodies are not produced

My treatment was killing my lymphocytes, which provide antibodies to fight infections and viruses. These are the cells which are enhanced to fight COVID-19 via the Pfizer and Moderna vaccinations. As a blood cancer patient, my lymphocytes are very low, thus COVID-19 antibody tests were used to test for the presence of antibodies after my vaccination, to check to see if the vaccination was working. These antibody tests provide critical information so risk can be managed and mitigated.

Scans deliver unexpected results

Scans may show unexpected good news! You may be quicker to remission or cure. Scans may also show your treatment is not working as expected. You will likely get scans during the treatment to evaluate the effectiveness of your treatment plan. Often, the scan is done halfway through the treatment cycle. If the treatment is not working, or working better than expected, you will know. After treatment, you will get a scan to confirm it worked, and then have more frequent scans in the first year or two—again, confirming all is A-OK. Each cancer is different, but expect the first five years post-cancer to include scans. Some cancers require frequent scans for the rest of your life.

Unexpected things will happen, so be mentally ready for the unexpected.

Appointments are re-scheduled

The unexpected can also mean missing appointments or tests for reasons out of your control. For example, I had to miss appointments during two hurricanes. And of course, the COVID-19 pandemic impacted my appointment schedules.

Care team changes

You may have to change your care team for various reasons. Also, don't be surprised if a key person on your care team either changes teams or leaves completely. At a large treatment center, the replacement care team member will be great, too.

Buddy changes

Sometimes, your buddy can't go with you as expected. Your buddy may get sick, or perhaps they have a conflict that prevents them from going with you to an appointment. You will need to find a replacement.

Insurance issues

Insurance may impact where you can get treatment. In the US, you can apply for continuation of coverage in order to be able to remain where you are being treated under a change to your insurance plan. There are times, too, when insurance won't cover a scan.

Your attitude and emotions change

You may be surprised by changes in your attitude and your emotions. There is a cumulative emotional and mental impact of going through cancer treatment. Emotionally and mentally, it gets harder, not easier. A friend once asked me, "Bill, do you have anxiety from your cancer battle?" I pondered it and then answered, yes, I do have times when it is a bit overwhelming, and I get anxious. My wife asked me this question the other day: "Are you scared to be around people?" I replied that I am scared to be around people because I am afraid of getting sick. Of beating the cancer but losing to the flu or COVID-19. I am scared my weakened immune system will cause me to die.

Every single time I go for a CT or PET scan the stakes are high. Waiting for the results is getting harder. I have heard "your cancer is back" too many times. But many more times I have heard, "you are still in remission." But dammit, each time it is getting harder to walk into the building for the test. Harder to sit with the doctor to hear the results. Harder to sleep the night before the tests or the results.

13

DYING AND THE ODDS

EARLY IN my journey, I tried not to contemplate death too often. By cancer number four, though, I decided I had better get my head around the idea of dying. Who was I kidding? Not only was the cancer a risk, but the risks from the treatment, the side effects, and the compromised immune system were serious. In 2014, just months after my treatment finished, I went to church, sat by a sick person, and promptly got pneumonia. That was an eye opener. My poor body could not fight or beat the pneumonia until a heavy dose of antibiotics was administered.

So how do you get your head around the possibility of dying? This was without a doubt the most difficult chapter in the book to write. How do you share with other cancer patients the best way to deal with thoughts of dying, knowing that each person and journey is unique? A goal of this book is to provide help and hope for those going through cancer treatment. But, if this is a book about cancer uncut—how can I not address death and dying? After all—the title of the book is *Up for the Fight*—fighting to beat cancer. I have been fighting to live for twenty years, advocating for myself so I don't die. I know, too, that my cancer is coming back and that getting to my goal age of ninety-three will take a lot of miracles. I would be deceiving myself if I did not think about it. NOT thinking about it would be mentally and emotionally unhealthy.

I am not an expert and struggle myself with thoughts of dying. I often wonder, is it wrong to think about dying? Will these thoughts impact my ability to heal? How do I have a conversation with my family about it? What is the right age to have a discussion about death with my kids? Can they handle it? What about friends and family—is it too much of a downer to talk about death with them?

All I can do is provide some thoughts based upon my personal experience.

Yes, you need to think about it. You don't want to be surprised by death. Those last days are not the time to try and get your head around it. Accept that it happens. It was healthier for me to confront the possibility of dying versus hiding it inside of me. This does not mean I am fighting any less hard. It is not a weakness to think about it. I don't obsess about my own mortality. I rarely talk about it. But I do think about it.

Yes, you should discuss it with your spouse or partner. They need to know how you feel and they, too, need to think about it and plan, as opposed to being surprised later. Denial by a spouse or partner of the seriousness of cancer is not uncommon. Conversations about death and dying are challenging, and can be very hard on your spouse or partner. I avoided it for a long time. This is a good opportunity to lean on professional help to gain insight on how to approach the subject. As addressed in Chapter 7, on the business of cancer, it is also important to have legal paperwork, like a will, prepared and handled in advance.

Talking to your children about the possibility you might die? It depends. It depends on their age and their maturity.

It is more than just getting your affairs in order. **It is important to get your head and heart in order, too.**

Each situation is different. Was it right to never talk about it with my young kids? Maybe. Would they have been shocked and surprised if I died while they were young? Yes. Once they got out of high school, was it OK to discuss with them? Probably.

Do I talk to friends about it? Rarely, except for a few close friends. And for them, the brutal honesty was hard, but little really had to be said. They already knew.

Here is my advice. Confront it. Accept the reality that it could happen. Don't obsess about it—but don't do like I did for years, and avoid it. And you do need to talk about it with someone, ideally a professional. Not in the "consume your life" way, but in the "it is healthy to think about it so I have thought about it and am prepared if it happens" way. Your spouse/partner and support team need to discuss the potential of your death, too, just in case. It is more than just getting your affairs in order. It is important to get your head and heart in order, too.

Pondering dying forces a reset as to how you view the world. How you view life. How you view living. I live a better life because of my bouts with cancer. Not the physical part, that has been and is a mess and I suffer way more than my fair share. But the better life is due to my clear perspective.

Yes, my attitude is usually, but not always, good. My care team is great. My support team is great. But sometimes, the ball just bounces the wrong way and death happens. I know how it can happen. I have seen it happen. And I am keenly aware of that possibility.

Why am I not afraid of dying? Because I know where I am going when I die. Heaven. Through my Christian faith, I know it. I spend quiet time with God every morning.

Praying for others but also praying for the care team. I rely on His direction. His presence. Your faith or spirituality might give you comfort as well.

I know too, that if I die, I have given beating cancer 100 percent of my effort and done my best. I can hold my head high and know that I fought a great fight. That I left no stones unturned. That I owned the journey. That I had the right team. That I did everything I could to live, and while living, I lived with purpose and care. That I help change lives. With a positive attitude. With heart. That I used my journey to help and inspire others.

This is also why I am conflicted about being called a cancer survivor. It sounds like an honor that I don't deserve. I have lived. So far. Why celebrate me surviving when others have not? But I know surviving should be celebrated. Call yourself what you want, but celebrate when you beat your cancer.

Let your friends and family and care team celebrate it, too. Smile when they call you a survivor.

The odds don't count

In my twenty-year cancer journey I have only had this question asked to me once—by an acquaintance who lived nearby—but it stuck with me. "Bill, what are your odds?" Holy cow. I had just had another surgery, another cancer diagnosis, and THIS is the question he chose to ask. I was shocked, saddened, and furious all at the same time. This is literally the worst question I have ever heard related to cancer. Why?

The ODDS don't count.

I tell people my odds are 100 percent. Then I let it sit. I say nothing.

Pause.

I look them in the eye as they think about it. I nod my head.

Most get it after about five seconds and have an "aha!" moment and nod their head in understanding. "Yes, I get it."

If they still don't understand my point, I prompt them again.

"My odds are 100 percent."

It is 100 percent certain that I will either live or die from the cancer. Period. There is no 50 percent.

If the written "odds" are one in a million to beat my type and stage of cancer—and I do beat it—I have 100 percent lived.

If your doctor wants to discuss odds, ask whether it really needs to be discussed, or tell your doctor you would prefer not to know the odds. There are only a few reasons to tell any patient odds based upon history—history with patients who are not you.

But, like me, many of you will want to look it up. If you do, remember: the odds don't count. So, if you look it up, read it and forget it.

Improved treatments

Cancer treatments are advancing so rapidly that with many cancers, any data out there regarding survival rates is irrelevant. Take lung cancer as an example. Historically, lung cancer has accounted for a large percentage of cancer deaths. However, lung cancer treatment advances have happened so fast that there are no accurate data on five-year (or more) survival rates. But we do know that the treatments are working better than ever. Advances are dramatically improving outcomes with many other types of cancers, too. Here are a few of many examples of rapidly advancing technologies:

- Messenger RNA or mRNA. Synthetic genetic codes to make proteins. This is the same technology used to create some of the most effective COVID-19 vaccines. Most of us heard about mRNA for the first time during the pandemic—but it has been known and researched for cancer treatments for a long time. Over time, expect success with mRNA.

- CRISPR or genome-editing technology. There is a great book on this topic, Walter Isaacson's *The Code Breaker*. CRISPR technology is already being tested to treat sickle cell anemia and is being studied for treating and curing a wide range of cancers. The first cancer clinical trial in the US was in 2019—so while researchers are hopeful, a lot of work still needs to be done.

- The BiTEs method from Amgen. My care team is researching this method as a potential future treatment for my lymphoma.

- CAR T-cell therapy.

- Immunotherapy continues to be a successful development in the treatment of cancer. Expect more breakthroughs here.

So, whatever your type of cancer, expect big, positive changes moving forward.

This is why I tell people, the longer I live, the longer I *will* live. Advances are happening at an exponential rate.

Miracles do happen. Results that defy expectations. Things that can't be explained. And there are many little miracles that can happen throughout the journey. So be ready for them!

14

ADVICE FOR FAMILY AND FRIENDS

A s THE patient, it is important to be aware of and respond to how your family is handling your cancer journey. Increase communication with them. Ask them how they are doing. Be aware of any changes in mood or behavior, so you can get them help, if needed. Keep an eye on their grades at school. Or their performance at work. It is easy to assume they are OK and handling it well, but with 100 percent certainty, they are not 100 percent OK. Be open to providing them resources and support to help guide them through it. Don't forget, they are in the Cancer Club now, too.

My wife has been dealing with my cancer journey for the majority of our marriage. My three kids have grown up with it. I can't imagine the burden this has put on them. But they have learned a lot from it.

Insight from my wife, Kim Potts

Being the spouse of a cancer patient once is tough; being the spouse of a cancer patient six times is even tougher!

When Bill was first diagnosed with thyroid cancer, the treatment seemed straightforward with a good prognosis.

You must take care of yourself so you can best help your cancer-fighting spouse.

The diagnosis of lymphoma, though, changed the complexion of the disease for me. Due to the age of our children and our desire to keep their lives as normal as possible, I did not travel with Bill to Houston from our home in Tampa for most of the lymphoma treatments. He stayed with his parents, who were very caring, at their home in Houston.

Looking back, I would have been with him each day for every hour of his treatment. It is so important, for his sake and mine, to make sure all is going right with the treatments. Was he getting enough to drink? Was anyone walking with him to the restroom? Was he cold? Hot? Hungry? The staff at both hospitals where Bill has been treated have been attentive to his needs, but this is never the same as having a loved one nearby.

As the spouse of a cancer patient, especially for one with multiple encore performances, you have to deal with the practical and emotional side of your loved one's care. Bill has always been on top of his medications and treatment plan, but an equally important part of beating cancer is attitude. Bill has always been a positive, "can do" type of person. He approached cancer the same way.

HOWEVER, THIS last time was a bigger hill to climb. Bill needed more pushing and pulling to get to the top of the hill. You have to remind your spouse constantly that this battle will be won. Don't let them see you sweat. If you believe your spouse can beat anything, then everyone around you will believe it, too.

You must take care of yourself so you can best help your cancer-fighting spouse. My main diversion throughout Bill's cancer treatment is to play tennis two, three, sometimes four times a week! It is good exercise, but more importantly, my friends are a source of comfort and support for me. Bill asks me if I won, and some days I have to really think about it, because the time spent on the court is about more than just the game.

I always make time for a daily devotion and spend time every day in what the pastor of our church describes as "the quiet place." This time helps me get a breath of fresh air from the day-to-day shadow of cancer and remember that a higher power is helping us get through it.

There are many emotions that rise to the surface when your spouse is fighting cancer. Aside from the fear of the loss of your "other half," there was, for me, also anger, sadness, frustration, and gratefulness.

The fear is not just for your loved one, but for yourself as well. If something happens to you, what will happen to your spouse, or all the other people who are relying on you to keep things going while your spouse is fighting cancer? The weight of that responsibility is heavy. It feels like everything is falling on you.

The sadness of seeing your spouse go through the process of treatment is difficult, knowing that all you can do is pray and love them.

There is a very real frustration, for me, at having to go through the process over and over again. We are supposed to be doing other things at this stage in our lives. How many times does he have to go through cancer treatment? Why can't it just go away and stay away?

But I also experience the gratefulness for all that we have been given despite having to fight this battle, again. Grateful for the excellent medical care, grateful for our friends who fly in to see us just to see firsthand that Bill is doing OK. The constant calls, emails, visits, and fabulous food and gifts our friends provide us put a smile on our faces.

Lastly, I am grateful for our children. When we started this journey of battling cancer we tried to protect them from what Bill was going through. Now, they are a source of strength for both of us. Now, we let them help us.

Be aware of your emotions and do something about them, so that you do not become a casualty from the fall-out of this disease.

Insight from my daughter, Anna Potts

My dad has had cancer for twenty of my twenty-four years. He has been diagnosed with cancer six times. His cancer is my normal.

I can't offer a one-size-fits-all approach for how you support a parent with cancer, but I will offer suggestions that may set you on the right path and put you in the right mindset.

If you're planning on being part of your parent's support system, be sure to have your own. I have found support through friends, family, faith, community, and even therapy. You can only give out of what you have, so have support!

You may want to be a rock for your family. But please be sure to take care of yourself. Having a parent with cancer is challenging in many ways. It shifts the parent-child care paradigm—they will inevitably rely on you more. You may also suddenly be confronted with the idea of mortality, and that is a huge can of worms! Take the time and space you need to process what is going on around and within you. You will find yourself more equipped to journey forward with your family, and perhaps even better equipped to live a fuller life.

Be encouraging. Sometimes encouragement sounds or feels cliché, but cancer patients need it. For me this looked like a quick phone call before a full day of treatment just to tell him he could do it.

Stay in touch! I had a conversation with my parents when my dad's cancer came back in 2020 about my plans to move from Florida to Boston, Massachusetts. I had planned to move right when my dad would begin treatment. I wondered, should I still go? My parents encouraged me to follow through with my move. I did, and while I cannot see them as often in person (especially in the era of COVID-19), we text, FaceTime, and talk on the phone. Make an effort wherever you are. Wherever you find yourself, don't be afraid to ask your parent how you can best support them. Similarly, help out when and where you're needed.

Keep a good attitude, but if you can't manage to, don't let it rub off on your sick parent.

Be intentional. Somehow, when cancer rears its ugly head, it forces you to be intentional. Allow it to positively transform how you approach your relationships with loved ones. Small acts of intentionality are the best because they are so accessible. For example, my twin sister, Sarah—my other half, who is incredibly thoughtful and intentional, a true caretaker—picks up a popsicle for Dad every time she gets off work on the weekends.

Recognize that your presence may mean more than anything eloquent you could try to say or do. Please do

Recognize that your presence may mean **more than anything eloquent you could try to say or do.**

not tell them how they should feel ("aw, don't be sad!"), and please do not also "reframe" their situation with statements like "it could be worse." This lacks tact and sensitivity, and often hurts. Listen, empathize, and if you do not have the words, your presence will likely mean more anyways. I remember clearly one of the days my dad came home from treatment for a relapse of his lymphoma when I was a senior in high school. He was wearing a purple dress shirt, tucked in neatly, and his hair—a full head of it that he has amazingly been able to keep—was well-trimmed. He looked sharp, but weary. He walked in the door, greeted us, sat in one of the living room chairs, and cried. It was one of the first times I truly saw him break down. I don't remember us saying much at all, but rather just being there. That's what truly counts.

Insight from my son, Nick Potts

There's one fact everyone knows but no one expects to face at a young age. Your parents will die.

My dad has had cancer nearly my entire life and for most of his cancer journey the possibility he may pass away from his illness was in the far back of my mind. Many families do face hardships with the early loss of a parent but the reality is most people don't think it will happen to theirs.

At twenty-six, in the height of a pandemic, and with my dad facing an increasingly serious treatment regimen, it hit me crystal clear that in eight months I might be the sole male Potts left in the bloodline. My dad assured me that the family lawyer would tell me everything I needed to know about managing his remains and the myriad of processes that kick in when a person dies. Let me tell you, that's an awful conversation to have.

It's easy for this harsh reality to consume you while watching your parent or loved one undergo a cancer treatment regimen, but it doesn't have to be that way. Here's how I found some peace through the process:

1   The stats don't matter. Stop Googling everything. Immediately. Whatever WebMD says survival rates are is irrelevant to you. Your parent or loved one will have a situation unique to them, their health, and their treatment plan, and fixating on the stats made up of thousands of other patients will simply not matter much. I didn't look at the survival stats for my dad's version of lymphoma until after the third time he had it. The only statistic that matters is their own.

2   Trust the system. Given the title of the book, I'll caveat this by reminding the reader that self-advocacy is important here as well. Oncologists are some of the most highly trained medical professionals in the world, as are the surgeons that operate on certain types of cancer patients. Cancer treatment is complicated but very well researched and understood. Medicine continues to improve and treatments are increasingly customizable to the patient. Cancer treatment and its side effects are also temporary, and treatment is frequently successful. Trust your medical professionals; they know what they're doing.

3   Take advantage of time. Throughout my dad's cancer journey, I understood the importance of spending time together. I didn't always grasp his mortality but a part

of me knew staying close to him was important given his history with cancer. Spend time with your parent while they go through treatment. Sit on the patio and talk about anything and everything. If they're healthy enough or in remission, go for walks, trips, or out to eat with them whenever you can. If you're far away, call them a few times a week. Some of the best memories I have with my dad were fueled by the fact we didn't know when he'd get cancer again, so we lived for the present. Part of why I rarely focused on my dad's mortality is because I have a great relationship with him. If he died, I'd regret little. This doesn't mean obsess over spending time with your parent, but prioritize extra time with them. That evening back in town catching up with friends? Maybe it can wait. Your friends will still be there, your parent may not be.

4   Live your life. Perhaps this point is more controversial in the broader context, but live your life. Seriously. Your life will change when a parent gets cancer, but keep the routines, hobbies, and work schedule you had, to at least some extent. This will help maintain a sense of normalcy and purpose and keep your mind from fixating on the heavier side of what cancer treatment can be. This is why I recommend prioritizing extra time for your parent, but not obsessing over them. Your life matters too and it's completely OK, healthy in fact, to keep moving forward for yourself.

The most important thing is to build a good relationship with your parent or loved one undergoing cancer treatment. It's OK to be shaken, upset, and depressed about a cancer diagnosis. As you process things, remember that shaken, upset, and depressed are not the only ways to feel. Maintaining a strong relationship with your cancer patient is the easiest way to find solace where it seems there could never be any.

Considering these points will hopefully help ensure that if the worst comes now or years in the future, you will be stronger and ready to tackle the hardest days of your life with a little more grace.

Lastly, cancer treatment WORKS and can work for your cancer patient.

Advice for friends: Back to Bill

Beating cancer is a team effort and your friends are a critical part of the support team for a cancer patient. Your friends are a part of your Cancer Club, too. This section is dedicated to all the friends of cancer patients, with the goal of helping them be a better friend to their friend battling cancer.

Friends, many times, are at a loss about what to do when they have a friend with cancer. I have had friends who were so uncomfortable that they just disappeared, and I heard nothing from them. I don't take this personally. I understand that my having cancer can bring up deep emotions in them. Maybe from personal experience. Maybe from fear. For some, the best way to handle it is to avoid it.

Most friends don't fall into this camp, though. They want to help you and be a part of your team.

But first, advice for you, the patient. Let them help you. Practice the art of saying "yes" when a friend offers to help you. Allowing them to help you helps them!

What not to say or do
. . . .

Do not ask the patient "what are your odds?" We have discussed this one already. The odds don't count.

Please don't tell a patient that they will "beat cancer." You don't know and while you may mean this to be encouraging, it is not. It is a throwaway comment—meant to make you, the friend, feel better, not the patient.

Please don't tell a patient they will "beat it because of their great attitude." Again, this is not true. I have known many patients who make my positive attitude and faith seem small. And they have lost their battle. This comment also falls in the camp of making you, the friend, feel better, not the patient. So just don't say it.

Do not tell the patient about your cancer, your friend's cancer, or anyone else's cancer. That shifts the focus away from the cancer patient—to you—or to someone else. Just focus on the patient. Talk with them about their cancer, if they even want to talk about it. You may mean well but are inadvertently shifting the focus to yourself and away from your friend.

Pretty please, don't cry when you visit a cancer patient. The patient is the one who should be crying. If you cry, the patient is compelled to comfort you. Here we go again, the conversation shifts from your friend to you. Most of my friends, when they come over to see me, are wondering what I will look like. But rarely do they cry at seeing me. Thank goodness!

Don't recommend a doctor or cancer treatment center without being asked. If your friend, the cancer patient, asks, tell them what you know. But if not, don't make a recommendation. Choosing a care team is a very personal decision. Just support them in it. It is A-OK to ask them where they are going and who is treating them. Just don't question it or suggest somewhere else for them to go.

Do not tell the patient about or recommend treatments you have heard or read about unless they ask. Trust the patient to be doing their homework. From medicine used to treat animals, to going to other countries for treatment, to drinking a special juice, to eating a special diet—you may have heard about many. Just leave these conversations for the patient to have with their care team.

Never, ever, ever, ever, ever go see a cancer patient if you are not feeling well or if you have had close contact with someone who is ill. Assume the patient is immuno-compromised, and a common cold could be life threatening. One hundred percent of the time, they will be appreciative if you call them and tell them you can't come over because you don't want to risk getting them sick. With COVID-19 and the flu, this becomes even more important.

My neighbors Jon and Amy are the best. They have been super supportive and thoughtful during my most recent battle. On more than one occasion they did not come over, even though we always see them outside, because one of them was not feeling great or they had been around someone who was sick. If you are not well, use Zoom, FaceTime, or an old-fashioned phone call to catch up instead of putting your friend at risk. Remember, if the cancer patient gets sick, they could die.

Do not ask the patient too many details about their cancer journey. It is hard to go through treatment, let alone talk about it.

Give your friend **the option of *not* talking about cancer.**

Do not bring your favorite home-cooked meal over to them. This tip was a source of disagreement even in our home. Food can be challenging for the patient. Sometimes things taste different. Sometimes food affects your stomach in odd ways. Sometimes you crave certain foods, like pregnant people do. Instead of bringing over your favorite home-cooked meal, ask your friend about a couple of their favorite restaurants. Then, ask them what they like at those restaurants. Order something from the restaurant, pick it up, and deliver it to them. You will make their day! This does not happen to me enough. (Hello, everybody! I love Chick-fil-A.)

What to do

Give your friend the option of *not* talking about cancer. Some of my best conversations while I was undergoing treatment were when my friends came over and talked about everything *but* cancer.

Do bring suggestions on ways they can spend any spare time. Funny movies, TV series, documentaries. Bring them books or magazines you think would be interesting for them to read.

Be understanding if your friend, the patient, is acting a bit irritable.

Be understanding if they forget something you have just told them or stumble over simple facts. As discussed, chemo brain is real. Jon and Amy were over on our patio one night when another neighbor, Mario, came over and asked me if it was OK to take our dog, Pippa, to their house to play. I agreed to it. Pippa loves them! Five minutes later

I yelled "where is Pippa?" Jon calmly answered, "She is at Mario's house." No sarcasm. No laughing. No, "don't you remember?" A perfect way to handle it. I was mad at myself at first for forgetting, but then remembered I forget a lot during chemo.

A GREAT thing you can do for your friend

Ask them, the patient, what they think they might like you to do to help and then suggest a few things you think they would enjoy. Thanks, Laurie L., for this tip! Once you hear their answer, pick something. Then—DO IT! That is true friendship. It might be as simple as walking their dog. Or taking them for a drive. Or listening to music with them. Or watching a sporting event with them. One of my personal favorites—an acquaintance, not even a close friend, asked me if he could take me fishing. "Yes," I said. "Please take me fishing!" Two days later, he did! Years later, I still remember it! Booyah!

The BEST thing to do

Tell your friend, the patient, you love them. This means more than anything else. I found that cancer shifted the paradigm with my friends. Before cancer, I would not tell my friends I loved them. It seemed odd. Now as a Cancer Club member, if I love them, I tell them. Then they tell me they love me, too! This has been amazing and special. So, tell your friend you love them. Make their day! They will make yours, too!

15

LOOK FORWARD AND KEEP GOING

N 2011, three years after being diagnosed with my first lymphoma, I raced and completed the IRONMAN Texas triathlon. I wanted to prove to my kids that anything is possible. There were a lot of reasons for me not to race. I was not the same person physically as I had been before the cancers. I had torn a ligament in my foot while training, and had not had sufficient time to train on running. Believe it or not, I removed a boot cast when training for the swim and trained on the bike throughout my recuperation. There were days I would ride 100 miles on the bike just to train. Then, I would put my cast back on.

The 2.4-mile swim at IRONMAN Texas started as the sun came up. I finished the 112-mile bike ride after three in the afternoon. As I changed into my running shoes after the bike ride, it was really, really hot. Like 100 degrees plus heat index hot. As I was about to start the marathon part of the race, my friend David B. asked me, "Bill, are you going to finish the race?"

Yes, I said, I had a plan—and would finish. All I had to do was run 26.2 miles—one mile at a time. And I did. I ran one mile to each aid station, drank, put ice in my shirt and shorts and then ran another mile to the next aid station. I ran one mile, twenty-six times.

At 8:41 pm that night—or thirteen hours and forty-one minutes after I started—I crossed the IRONMAN finish line, and as my family hugged me, I knew they had learned that anything is possible. My son has followed in my footsteps and completed two IRONMAN 70.3 events.

I learned so much from this event that applies to the cancer journey, such as:

- Set smaller short-term goals while working toward a bigger one.

- Tune out pain to help achieve your goals. The pain will likely diminish.

- Anything is possible through hard work and focus.

- Be patient as you pursue your goal.

- The unexpected happens, so be ready for it, plan for it, and adapt.

Your big goal is to beat cancer. Break this down into a lot of small goals. Then, celebrate those small goals. Getting the port installed. Completing the first treatment. Getting to the halfway point of treatment. These are all milestones that will get you to the finish line. Achieve them, let out a booyah, and savor it.

Count the treatments. Count up until you get to the halfway point—and then count down until you finish. For example, for my fourteen days of chemotherapy and immunotherapy infusions with my most recent lymphoma treatment, I counted up to seven. One infusion complete. Two infusions complete. When I got to number seven, I celebrated that I was halfway finished. Too early to ring the

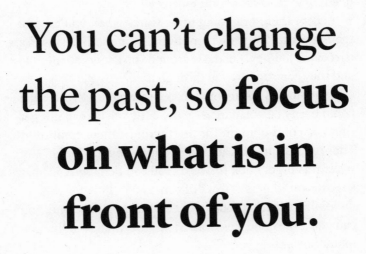

You can't change the past, so **focus on what is in front of you.**

bell—but I was so happy! Then, I started counting down. Six infusions to go. Five infusions to go and so on until I completed my treatments. This counting process helped me stay positive. I was tracking my progress and making progress!

Recognize and appreciate other victories along the way. For me, the first night I was able to sleep through the night after a treatment was a cause for joy. I would wake up and tell my wife, "I slept!" Walking around the block without needing to rest was another victory!

Accept there are going to be times when you are not feeling well. Physically, emotionally, mentally. This is a part of the journey. Let those around you know your mood—and they can support you through it.

Don't look back at your journey; always look forward. I could easily be consumed by my early mistake in not getting a second opinion for my thyroid cancer treatment. That mistake has created challenges beyond belief. But resist this urge. Look forward. You can't change the past, so focus on what is in front of you.

Joining support groups will help you not feel alone. You can get some good tips from them, too, on how to handle many cancer issues.

Be a patient patient. This not only helps your care team but will help you maintain a positive attitude.

Daily exercise, even walking, can boost your spirits.

Eating well makes you feel better, which will help your attitude.

Staying away from depressants like alcohol will also help.

Practice smiling. It works to make your attitude better and the attitude of those around you better!

Helping others will help you stay positive. These can be cancer patients you mentor, or just volunteering your time to help others.

Don't let cancer prevent you from living. Do whatever you feel you can do during your journey. If you can carve out time before treatment to visit a park near the treatment center—do it. If you can stay at a hotel on the beach during treatment. Do it. Do those things that make you happy. With cancer, those things may change, but be deliberate in trying to experience life.

BE GRATEFUL for those who are helping you. Your family, friends, your care team, and all the others who support you.

Never stop managing your battle

My dad's brother and my namesake, Bill Potts, a US Army soldier, was killed in action just before the end of World War II. While I knew a lot about Bill from a book his dad had written about him, it was rare that my dad spoke about him. One day, I was curious and asked my dad, "Dad, how often do you think about your brother Bill?" His answer surprised me. "Oh, I think about him every day."

It is this way with cancer, too. You may have finished your journey, but you will not forget it. There is not a day that goes by that I don't think about cancer. For me, that starts every morning when I take the pill that tries to substitute for the hormones I don't get from my missing thyroid.

Each day, while I am grateful for all my blessings, including beating cancer, I am troubled by what may come. We still must handle my prostate cancer and I know my

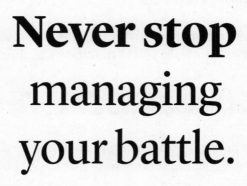

Never stop
managing
your battle.

lymphoma will be back. The prospect of the recurrence of my lymphoma, frankly, scares me, as I know that beating cancer number seven will be more challenging and difficult.

Even if your cancer is cured, you, too, will think about it potentially coming back. If you don't think about it every day like me, you will think of it often. Every ache and pain, sickness, lump, or any other changes to your body will put you on high alert. Before cancer, a cold was a cold. A lump in your neck was a swollen lymph node, due to the body working its magic to heal you. Now, though, you wonder if your cancer is coming back. You may wonder too, in the case of a second or third cancer, whether a newly diagnosed cancer may have been caused by your previous cancer or previous cancer treatments.

Once in the Cancer Club, you need to be vigilant about your body.

If you have ANY concerns, confer with your medical care team. Let them know. Determine the cause. Get ahead of it, just in case. You will likely be able to cut the line to quickly get any of these issues reviewed by your care team.

Continue to advocate for yourself. Continue to be focused on your body. Don't let your guard down.

Never stop managing your battle.

Your life depends on it.

Decide your type

There is a bell curve of the types of cancer patients I have known. Most of the patients, or the middle of the bell curve, approach it as an important part of their lives, a focus of their lives, but they do not let it define them. They own it and manage it like a job. They fight it calmly. They are not the same person as before—they have been changed by the cancer—but they move on. The Pragmatists.

Some deny it or just give up after the diagnosis; for whatever reason, they are not up for the fight. The Deniers.

Some let cancer define them. What they say and do revolves around cancer. They become known to all as the "cancer patient." Or the "cancer survivor." The Definers.

You get to decide your type.

Always have hope

I focus on hope by looking at the positive, not the negative. I learned a lot about hope when working at Clearwater Marine Aquarium. Hope is an orphaned dolphin who was rescued when she was two months old by the same team who rescued the famous Winter, the dolphin who survived without a tail. Winter learned to swim with a prosthetic tail and was made famous by the 2011 movie *Dolphin Tale*.

Hope arrived at the aquarium on the night of the last day of filming for *Dolphin Tale*. Incredibly, Hope survived, became friends with Winter, and is the basis for the fantastic real-life sequel, *Dolphin Tale 2*. I spent a lot of time with Winter and Hope and was inspired by their stories, as were millions of others. Winter and Hope both surviving. Both living together. The odds were almost zero. Their story proves that miracles happen and there is always hope.

LAGNIAPPE

WENT TO college in New Orleans at Tulane. While there, I learned some great things about Cajun culture. One of those was *lagniappe* (pronounced lan-yap)— meaning a bonus or something extra. Well, I have learned more than I expected during my cancer battles, so will share some *lagniappe*.

You have made it this far in the book and learned about advocating for yourself and how to navigate the cancer journey. Like you, I ponder how cancer has changed me. I accidently became a cancer expert and cancer accidently changed me in profound ways.

If you are finishing your treatments, I highly recommend that you ring the bell that is provided for patients to ring after their last infusion or radiation treatment. For me, I know I will be back to get more chemo someday— but for now, finishing this part of the journey deserves a celebration. Ring the bell not just for you, but as a way of recognizing the efforts of your care team. It means a lot to them! So, ring the bell with them, and ring it with gusto!

Sometimes though, the fight won't be won. Despite all the efforts, the bell won't get rung. If that is your situation, then fight as hard as you can to inspire others in their fight. So that they can face their battle with the same level of courage and dedication that you did. Help them be up for the fight, by your example, so that hopefully, one day, they can ring the bell.

As you move forward to the next phase of your life, apply the lessons of *why*. Early in your cancer journey you connected with your whys on beating cancer. Now, connect with your whys in other areas of your life. Use those whys as your motivation. A few years ago, I spoke to 400 high-level medical professionals at a major hospital system in Texas. I gave a speech about reconnecting with your why at work. I asked the question of the audience, "Why are you in the health care field? Why do you do what you do?" A hand went up, and a woman shared this story:

"When I was fourteen years old, my dad died due to medical mistakes at the hospital. I decided right then that I wanted to be in the medical field, to be able to make an impact and try to prevent those types of mistakes from being made on the fathers of other little girls." Tears started streaming down her face. I asked her, "What is your job at the hospital?" She answered, "Vice President of Quality Control." Silence. Then cheers erupted from the room.

Believe in yourself. I now know anything is possible—if you put your mind to it and work hard. If you own it! Live a full life outside of life as a cancer patient.

The process of setting a lot of small goals to achieve the big goals during your cancer treatment works in life, too. You can climb any mountain or race any race! Step by step.

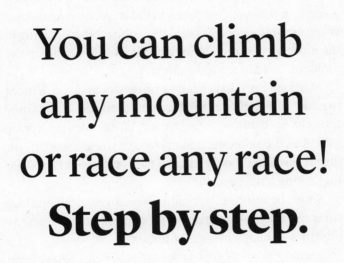

You can climb
any mountain
or race any race!
Step by step.

Live in the moment! Be present! Open your eyes so that you can see! There are millions of amazing things to see if you just look. That means ditching your phone, headphones, computer, often. When at dinner, engage in the conversations. And listen! When going on a walk—notice the beauty, smell the air, listen to the birds, watch the butterflies. Look up in the sky. When is the last time you looked up at the sky and tried to imagine what the clouds looked like? If you have not done it in a while—try it. When going to a concert, just listen to the music and soak it up. When at work—work. Focus. Live in the moment. Living in the moment also means not worrying while you are in the moment. Take in the today, today!

Make sure you have your priorities set and check them to make sure they are still the right priorities. Things may have changed during your journey. Write down your priorities. And then check in and make sure you are working on them. This book was a goal, and I am grateful to Page Two for making it happen.

Some of my best decisions have been making decisions on things NOT to do. Now, I spend my time on my priorities—and my life is a lot better.

Leaning into my faith has been life changing. I have been a part of many miracles and witnessed too many to count.

Focus more on taking care of yourself. Not only to be in good shape if the cancer comes back, but also to minimize the risk of getting another cancer. Do this by eating a healthy diet, exercising as often as you can, and making sure to allow time to rest. Take care of yourself better mentally, ensuring you have time to relax. Spend time on things you like and with people you care about.

Helping others works. As I dug deep going through my cancer battles, I learned that turning my thoughts outward to others, versus inward on myself, made me a lot happier and fulfilled. I am not the center of the world, but just part of it.

My friend Ben J. asked me the other day, "Bill, was it worth it? Was it worth having cancer?" I paused and thought about it before I answered, "For the first twenty years, no. Even though it changed me in so many positive ways. The suffering, the anxiety, the physical beatings, the stress, the impact on the family. I would not wish it on anyone. This book, though, is meant to help those in the Cancer Club. If it impacts one person, helps them in positive ways, helps them in their journey, then, yes, my journey will be worth it."

Thank you for reading this book. I hope it makes a difference.

Now, take what you learn during your journey and share it with another member of the Cancer Club. Turn your pain into purpose. And, like with me, this will make you happier and more fulfilled.

BOOYAH!

ACKNOWLEDGMENTS

BEATING CANCER and writing books are a team effort and I am fortunate to have an amazing team working with me on both.

My wife, Kim, and my three kids, Nick, Anna, and Sarah, have all been great and supportive and encouraging about this book, providing great thoughts and ideas for it.

Special thanks go to the MD Anderson and Mayo Clinic (Jacksonville campus) teams for continuing to save my life and providing great insights for this book. The staff of both were an open book with me, answering my many questions during my cancer journey. I learned so much from them. Thank you to Dr. Nathan Fowler, Liz Sorenson, Haleigh Mistry, Dr. Ernesto Ayala, Tammy McGarry, Jen Green, and pastor Tanya, who lit the fire for me to write this book, on the darkest day of my life.

Thanks too, to Page Two, the publisher of this book. This is not my book—but our book. They were there with me throughout battle number five, always providing me much needed encouragement. Those Friday afternoon

Zoom calls when we just laughed together were priceless. We even created two plans for the launch date (a new scenario for them). The first was if my health went south and the prognosis was that I would lose the battle; in that case, we would shift up the publication date. The second was the date should my treatments work. I am happy to report that we were able to go with the later publication date—I was up for the fight! Jesse Finkelstein, the co-founder of Page Two, is a great leader and a better person. Amazing Amanda Lewis is the best editor, writing coach, and mentor ever. Chris Brandt inspired me with his toughness. Adrineh Der-Boghossian kept me on track and on schedule, not an easy thing to do with a cancer patient! Jess Werb was a great help, too, supporting this book to the finish line! The Page Two team did not realize it when they started this journey with me, but now, they are a part of my Cancer Club. They are a blessing in my life. Because of their belief in the power of this book to help others, their belief in me to tell this story—my cancer journey is now worth it.

It would take a whole book to thank everyone else involved in my cancer and my book journey.

So, to all not named:

Thanks!

INDEX

ABOUT THE AUTHOR

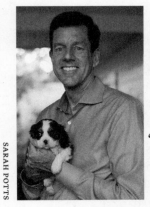

SARAH POTTS

BILL C. POTTS is a motivational speaker, creative business leader, energetic community builder, and dedicated father and husband. A five-time cancer survivor, he pursues life with the utmost passion and drive. While his kids say he's "sometimes slightly embarrassing," they also admit he's the "toughest man we have ever met." He loves his job and wakes up each morning expecting an A+ day—because every day is an A+ day, no matter the circumstances.

He has held executive positions at the IRONMAN Group and the Clearwater Marine Aquarium, and lectures on marketing at Tulane University, where he earned his MBA. He is the co-founder and a managing director of marketing agency Remedy 365 and an IRONMAN triathlete. He is a proud advisory board member of the Halo House Foundation, which provides affordable housing for cancer patients.

Bill lives in St. Petersburg, Florida, where he and his wife, parents of three adult children, owned a popular massage therapy franchise for fourteen years. His hobbies include playing tennis with his wife, Kim; walking his dog, Pippa; running; and reading. *Up for the Fight* is Bill's second book; he is also the author of the children's book *Ruby & Lizzie: The Raging River Adventure*, which he wrote for his twin daughters while they were at summer camp.

HELP THOSE IN THE CANCER CLUB

THANK YOU for reading this book. I am grateful to have had the opportunity to write it. I hope some of the lessons I have learned in my journey are helping you in your journey. Here's how you can help spread the word about this book, to help even more people:

- Provide a five-star review of this book on your favorite online retailer's website or reading community so that others can find and read it too. Those reviews make a big difference in so many ways. Thanks!

- Go to or send others to billcpotts.com for additional information and resources that will help in the cancer journey.

- Buy a copy (or give your copy) of *Up for the Fight* to someone you know in the Cancer Club!

- Follow me on my social media channels for updated Cancer Club information.
  🐦 @billcpotts
  📷 @billcpotts93
  📘 billcpotts

- Consider having me speak at your company or organization.

- Share your story with me at bill@billcpotts.com. It would be great to hear from you.